D1082863

The Future of Us

The Future of Us

*What the Dreams
of Children Mean to
Twenty-First-Century
America*

Irwin Redlener

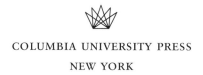

COLUMBIA UNIVERSITY PRESS

NEW YORK

Columbia University Press
Publishers Since 1893
New York   Chichester, West Sussex
cup.columbia.edu
Copyright © 2017 Irwin Redlener
All rights reserved

Library of Congress Cataloging-in-Publication Data
Names: Redlener, Irwin, author.
Title: The future of us : what the dreams of children mean to
twenty-first-century America / Irwin Redlener.
Description: New York : Columbia University Press, [2017] |
Includes bibliographical references and index.
Identifiers: LCCN 2017020979 (print) | LCCN 2017032107 (ebook) |
ISBN 9780231545945 | ISBN 9780231177566 (alk. paper)
Subjects: LCSH: Children—United States—Social conditions—21st century. |
Children—Government policy—United States. | Child welfare—
United States. | United States—Social conditions—21st century. |
United States—Social policy—21st century.
Classification: LCC HQ792.U5 (ebook) |
LCC HQ792.U5 R3445 2017 (print) |
DDC 362.70973—dc23
LC record available at https://lccn.loc.gov/2017020979

Columbia University Press books are printed on permanent
and durable acid-free paper.
Printed in the United States of America

Cover image: Provided by the author

For my kid brother Rick, who lit up our world, made us laugh, and helped us understand what it really means to love life.

Contents

Photo section follows page 130

Author's Notes
and Acknowledgments

I have tried, wherever possible, to keep the events recounted in this book chronological, though it wasn't always possible. In some cases it seemed more sensible to cluster certain stories under a topic heading, such as my experiences over the years with disasters.

I have also made liberal use of "representative dialogue," a technique commonly seen in memoirs. This is because very few of the conversations contained in the book were actually recorded or transcribed verbatim. In all cases, however, the dialogue as written does faithfully represent the absolute sense of the content, tone, and meaning of conversations that took place.

My final look at this manuscript occurred about six weeks after the inauguration of President Donald J. Trump. At that moment, the federal government seemed to be in a state of political chaos. This is never a good situation for vulnerable children and the people who advocate on their behalf. The Affordable Care Act and a host of safety-net programs were under threat of reduction or elimination. New directions for the federal Department of Education were also being discussed, as were potentially draconian new immigration policies. In essence, we were entering unchartered waters in terms of what low-income children and families could be facing. Time will tell. Perhaps by the time you read this we will know exactly what has been enacted, what has been fought back, and where we'll be going from here.

I have many people to thank, but let me start with the exceptionally talented and caring editors at Columbia University Press, Jennifer Perillo and Stephen Wesley. Their commitment to making this project happen was a tremendous source of encouragement throughout the entire process of making this book as good as it could be. And a special thanks to my agent, Steve Ross, who believed in this project from the beginning and helped make sure that we found a wonderful publisher.

Karen Redlener's support has been critical from start to finish. She turned out to be a spectacularly talented editor across the board, from content and tone, to verification of incidents described and recounted throughout the book, to copyediting. I don't think it would have been possible to bring this project to the finish line without her. I'm a lucky man!

A special thanks to the very talented Cory Sobel, a wonderful writer and researcher who was a pleasure to work with through all phases of this project.

My children Stephanie, Michael, and David have been incredibly supportive, with a special nod to Stephanie, who has been helping me come to grips with my eclectic career for years. And my appreciation and love to my grandchildren, Caleb, Mia, Naomi, Alia, Aaron, Sam, and Auren, constant reminders of why it all matters.

Finally, I am so very grateful to the many children and families whose stories are included in this book, and to the thousands who have taught me so much throughout my career. I am humbled by the millions of families who struggle with the severe adversities of poverty, confronting challenges few of us can imagine. And most of all, I think of the children who dream big, who aspire to the same life goals as my own grandchildren, and who deserve to have the pathways and possibilities for their lives wide open.

Irwin Redlener, MD
Cofounder, Children's Health Fund
Professor of Pediatrics
College of Physicians and Surgeons
Professor of Health Policy and Management
The Mailman School of Public Health
Columbia University
New York, New York

Foreword

For as long as I have known him—almost thirty years—I have believed that the story of the remarkable life and work of Dr. Irwin Redlener needed to be told. But *The Future of Us* is a revelation! I barely knew the half of it.

This is far more than the story of a doctor who has devoted himself to the care and well-being of vulnerable children. It is also about an activist who has fought for social justice since the early 1970s, using his MD to reach policymakers and elected officials where he has advocated for justice, fairness, and equal opportunity for every child in America. In the 1960s when President Lyndon B. Johnson declared a "war on poverty," Irwin Redlener signed up—and made it his life's mission.

What makes this book powerful is, in large part, the simplicity of Irwin's message: Too many children in America face adversities and disparities of opportunity that keep them from achieving their aspirations. This reality is terrible for the children who never fulfill their potential—and a disaster for the country as we enter a competitive, unpredictable future.

I can remember where I was when I first encountered Irwin's name. At home in the kitchen, my husband passed a newspaper article across the table at breakfast. It described a big blue mobile medical unit—picture a bus painted bright blue—a veritable doctor's office on wheels. Irwin was the doctor inside, making improbable "house calls" to the squalid transient hotels in midtown Manhattan. The hotels were ad hoc shelters for a city overwhelmed by the blight of homelessness, filled with destitute, despairing men and women.

New York's homeless problem was not news to anyone living there in the 1980s. I had a TV show that once featured a story about a man living on a fashionable block on Madison Avenue—in a box. And, of course, there were the so-called "bag ladies," pushing shopping carts, alone, so sad, so ubiquitous. But the revelation in the newspaper article that morning was the homeless *children*. They were all but invisible. It was unimaginable. But not to Irwin.

A child with no home has nothing. Maybe less than nothing if that child's caretaker is debilitated by the stress of poverty, compounded perhaps by addiction to drugs or abuse or neglect. Where to begin to solve that? Well, one very fundamental thing that child does not have is medical care. That's where Irwin stepped in. And where, a little later, I entered the picture. Within days of reading that newspaper article, a letter arrived for me at the *Today* show. I was a mother of three small children at the time, which made me doubly eager to say yes when Irwin asked if I'd lend my name to the advisory board of this young, ambitious, and innovative program called the Children's Health Fund. While I knew I had little advice of value to offer, how could I say no? And I've been privileged to be part of the mission ever since. Those small children of mine have started having kids now—it's been a long road.

So many children. The revelation of *The Future of Us* is just how many of the world's children Irwin *sees*. He's made it his life's mission to seek out children at greatest risk, finding the roots of his affinity in the vulnerability and sense of difference he felt in his own childhood. His life took a curious turn when as a child his family moved to rural Pennsylvania from Brooklyn and enrolled him in a one-room elementary school! As a young doctor in training, he took an internship at a hospital literally named Babies Hospital at Columbia Presbyterian Medical Center in New York City. There, so many of his patients had either arrived in the world too early or terribly sick or coming from the communities of profound poverty that surrounded the hospital. But Irwin has always been called by the most desperate cases—and sometimes causes— where only an optimist could find hope.

You'll follow him to a pocket of rural poverty in extremis in the deep south of still-segregated Lee County, Arkansas, in the 1970s. As an idealistic, long-haired doctor, a child of the Kennedy-Johnson era of social activism, he turns down a prestigious training program in pediatric cardiology and heads to Arkansas where he becomes director of a clinic run by the federal VISTA program (Volunteers in Service to America). He persevered despite being tailed by menacing white men in pickup trucks with gun racks, and was once awakened in the night to a burning cross in the yard. He was undeterred.

And at every step, Irwin dared to imagine that the great social ills of our country—racism, malnutrition, child abuse, poverty itself— were reversible! He was a product of his times, as we all are. I owed my seat at the anchor desk where Irwin found me to the sequence of the civil rights movement, the women's movement, and the less organized but no less profound "youth movement." These mass outpourings of rage and fairness were chaotic, noisy, paradigm-shifting and—sometimes—life-saving.

In 1985 a devastating famine in Africa awakened the world to the specter of mass starvation, and the stars came out. Do you remember USA for Africa and Michael Jackson's anthem, "We Are the World"? It was Irwin who was tasked with investing the outpouring of our donations to starving communities in Sub-Saharan Africa.

Which brings the story full circle. Back home in New York, one of those stars, singer-songwriter Paul Simon, was moved to action by a growing problem of homelessness in New York City. Joining forces with Irwin and Karen Redlener, the trio created the Children's Health Fund. From that first big blue bus to more than fifty mobile medical units today, CHF teams ply daily rounds in underserved, high-risk populations of children nationwide. And CHF advocates have been at the forefront of activists constantly fighting to sustain and expand the safety net programs needed by families and children still stuck in the cycle of poverty that has trapped so many Americans.

The Future of Us is a clarion call for another great movement. A children's movement. You'll find no pablum like "the children are our future." This is where the future begins; the future of us, our country, the world. It's past time, or as Irwin writes, "kids can't wait for complex adversities to be remedied." We need to eliminate these adversities now, for the sake of the children and to ensure a future of prosperity and success in the decades to come.

So, here finally is the story Irwin wrote: the memoir of an "activist pediatrician" who never had the time to pause and reflect about himself. But Irwin Redlener has never been too busy to find the time to do what was really important. And this book is exactly that.

And it's wonderful. Enjoy.

—Jane Pauley

Introduction

The Urgency of Childhood

I've raised four children, including a son who died in an accident—and I've loved every moment shared with our seven grandchildren, though the oldest of them endured and is recovering from a brain tumor. My son's death was an unspeakably tragic accident, my grandson's illness a terrifying encounter with an unavoidable disease.

But, unlike so many of the families I've seen in my career, I've never had a child or grandchild who will not be able to live a full and successful life because of barriers related to the income of his or her parents, the color of his or her skin, the gross inadequacy of his or her school, the inaccessibility of decent health care, or the consequences of heartless, shortsighted, or stupid government policies and spending priorities. These perspectives mark the core of my personal mission, based not on making every child "equal" but on the struggle to create equitable opportunity for all children to attain and sustain well-being.

Several of my grandchildren, including eight-year-old Naomi and fourteen-year-old Mia, asked me why I was writing this book about children, secretly hoping, I suspect, that they would be the central characters. They aren't, though it would be fair to say that my children and grandchildren—and yours—collectively have an enormous stake in the central questions this book explores and the challenges that need our urgent attention.

It boils down to this: Too many children in America (and around the world) live under conditions that threaten their abilities to achieve successful and fulfilling lives. This is an indisputable reality and a problem that, if left unresolved, reflects a moral failure to value and respect the aspirations of children and families. It also suggests a terrible misunderstanding of what it takes for any nation to remain economically viable and internationally influential.

During the 1970s, early in my career as a pediatrician and social justice advocate, America seemed deeply preoccupied with the overriding issues of the day, from the war in Vietnam to the toxic political environment of the Nixon administration. It never occurred to me that certain obvious truths about our basic values, like eliminating disparities and erasing all remnants of racism, would be such a hard sell in our nation—not here, where we still saw ourselves as the leading world power and the principal global purveyor of democracy, human rights, innovation, and economic strength.

Prior to the utter failure of America's military intervention in Southeast Asia and the big reveal about what was actually being perpetrated by Nixon and his administration, perhaps we allowed ourselves an inordinate level of national hubris that, looking back, seems, at the very least, naïve. We were struggling to understand, through a dense cloud of tragically misunderstood geopolitical realities and deliberate purveying of misinformation, what we were actually doing in Vietnam. We still bore the social wreckage of two centuries of American human and civil rights atrocities, and we still actively grieved the unbearable assassinations of John Kennedy, Robert Kennedy, and Martin Luther King, Jr.

But what has eluded me then and now—a half-century later—is why we still seem unable to understand what children need and how they perceive their own futures, and still seem incapable of making sure that every child has a reasonable pathway to a successful life.

Creating pathways for children to realize their dreams requires a clear understanding that every step of the process is fragile. On some level, this general understanding applies to every child, regardless of socioeconomic standing. It's just far less problematic when children are raised in environments of adequate resources, appropriate and timely access to needed services, and positive parenting strategies. It's not as dire even for children raised in poverty who happen to be inherently resilient, especially when internal resiliency is reinforced by a parent or other adult who can serve as a buffer against adversities that otherwise surround them.

But for all children, the laws of development are timely and essentially inviolate. From the moment of conception through adolescence, a varying combination of physical, biochemical, genetic, emotional, and stimulatory conditions affect the growth and development of a person's brain. The conditions at any given moment along the complex course of human development ultimately influence a person's capacity to think, function, process information, learn, and stay physically and psychologically healthy.

Once conceived, as the progression from embryo to fetus to viable infant unfolds over a typical 280-day course of pregnancy, the brain and nervous system, along with other body systems, organs, and physical dimensions begin to take shape as an array of controller genes mediates the precise order and pace of development.

The process continues in an orderly timeline, including in the first few years of life when brain growth is rapid and critical. Language absorption is key—and it must happen at a certain point in development if children are to be optimally ready for social interaction, reading, and comprehension at the appropriate times.

It is clear now that the number of words spoken to infants and toddlers of families living in extreme poverty are millions fewer than those typically heard through conversation and reading to babies and young children in more affluent households. This disparity makes a difference in learning readiness in early elementary grades. Healthy emotional and social development is also on the line. At certain moments of brain and neurological development, young children learn to "self-regulate" emotional responses and reactions to external and internal stimuli.

Once in preschool and through the early years of elementary education, the progression continues. Ideally, children are taught new skills at developmentally relevant points of readiness. There is an ideal window for learning to read, for instance, when the brain's readiness is at an optimal state. The same goes for developing computational skills.

It is worth remembering, too, that new skills build on those already acquired. Hearing words, lots of them and repeatedly, is a precursor to learning to read most efficiently. One step follows the next.

Nobody gets to be a paleontologist or a marine biologist without getting through middle school. People can't function in college if they don't reach an acceptable level of language and math skills via a successful high school experience. Peeling back a few layers, if children aren't prepared for kindergarten, they are likely not to be reading at grade level when they reach third grade. And that is an early indicator that graduating from high school on time is potentially unlikely.

No matter how poor and marginalized they may be, children dream and aspire. Our job, whether as parents, teachers, doctors, policy makers, or, I would say, voters, is to make aspirations *realizable* for every child. That's sometimes a very tough assignment in the inner cities or in the myriad of other communities in America's urban and rural "opportunity deserts."

This book is about why this is so and why failing to recognize and secure the aspirations and well-being of children may have irreversible consequences for America and the planet.

Yes, I know and fully appreciate that there are other, dire challenges facing our future. Drastic action to slow climate change, for instance, is for many people the first and foremost priority for every government on the planet. I don't argue with that. The hard truth is that securing a productive, safe, and peaceful future for the planet demands the capacity to deal with more than one challenge at a time.

Persistent racism, extraordinary poverty, epidemics of preventable disease, outbreaks of genocide, threats to planetary biodiversity, unfulfilled rights of women and members of the LGBTQ community, an unjust criminal justice system, the rise of violent terrorism, and a host of other challenges confront many other nations on the planet, from the most to the least developed. Each of these issues deserves intense focus and attention.

But what should be well understood is that the failure to secure the future of children, the inability to make sure they maximize their full potential, and a blasé unwillingness to do whatever it takes to provide a clear trajectory for every child to express and fulfill his or her aspirations will spell trouble for America by the middle of this century. This is because each child who does not reach his or her potential must live with serious challenges that could have been prevented or mitigated. These conditions lead to the need for remediation and, far too often, involvement in the criminal justice system. In many cases, there can be a measurable impact on lifelong productivity and aspirational fulfillment of adults who have had avoidable struggles from infancy though adolescence.

The statistics speak for themselves. For a child born today, the probability of a white male's ending up incarcerated is one in seventeen. But for a Hispanic male child, the chances are one in six, and, particularly disconcerting, a male African American infant born today has a one in three chance of ending up in prison.[1] And, as I discuss further later in the book, while high school graduation rates are generally improving and stand at more than 83 percent of all students in 2015, only 70 percent of black children graduate on time.[2]

There's another point worth mentioning. In order to get beyond slogans, political pandering, and clichés like "Children are our most valuable resource" or, my personal favorite inane fluffery, "Children are our future," we have to assume a far more specific strategic posture. Those who aspire to advance the prospects for children and family issues must leverage politics, public opinion, and resources with the persistence and urgency we regularly see on behalf of big pharma, the real estate industry, hospitals, and the like.

The work to ensure the health and well-being of children is serious, grown-up business. We need heartstrings to be tugged by the folks who work on the front lines of caring for children in need. We certainly need calls for compassion and charity. But we also need the hard-core, take-no-prisoners types who demand that those empowered to determine priorities and allocate resources understand and respond to the needs of children.

This book focuses on a single theme, an overriding societal goal: fulfilling the promises and potential of all children. My own life experiences have been eclectic, at times driven by serendipity and other forces I may or may not fully understand. But I have seen many children in many environments, too many under circumstances that not only threaten their potential development but actually threaten their literal survival.

That is why the work of protecting children involves a wide, some might say overwhelming, range of concerns, from children in poverty without access to decent health care or good education, to children who have been physically or psychologically abused, to children vulnerable during and after a major disaster, to those who end up in the pediatric intensive care units and those who might have needed advanced medical care where none was available.

Throughout the book you will be introduced to many of the children I have met in my work over the past four decades, but especially those I have encountered through the Children's Health Fund (CHF), the organization that Paul Simon and I, with the invaluable help of Karen Redlener, founded in 1987. CHF provides more than 260,000 health care visits each year, mostly in unique mobile child health clinics serving vulnerable children and families in some of America's most economically disadvantaged urban and rural communities. I think you'll understand why I love these children and the futures they envision, but fear the barriers that impede their abilities to achieve their perfectly reasonable dreams.

I should point out that while we will spend time getting to know some extraordinary children who dream big but face obstacles that seem—and, too often, actually are—overwhelming, we will also meet other children who make it through the challenges in spite of growing up with serious adversities.

In addition, this book shares some of my own—let's just call it like it is—"unusual" personal and professional experiences which, collectively, may shed some light on how I came to a point of chronic frustration about how long it's taking us to understand how important it is to care for children and their futures, yet still remain optimistic and energized about what can and will be done going forward. I'll leave it to you to decide if having dinner with Fidel Castro before touring Cuba's health care system, sitting across the table from Michael Jackson as he ranted about a song he didn't write, or traveling with presidential candidates on the campaign trail is relevant to the bigger story about children and their prospects for a well-lived life in America.

I do know that the years spent practicing medicine in a poverty-stricken, racially torn Southern county and in the homeless shelters of New York City, and my work with badly abused children and those caught up in terrible natural disasters, have added, one after another, to my personal gestalt—every experience in some way irrevocable and contributing to my particular take on our societal priorities.

One of the biggest challenges in writing this book was figuring how, perhaps why, to include the autobiographical elements found herein. I felt from the outset that understanding something of my own roots would help me understand for myself, if no one else, what made me so driven to deal with inequities, with social justice, with persistence in the face of adversity. So I went back to some very early experiences that ultimately helped define my worldview as I found my way into adulthood. It was, in fact, these accumulated experiences—in childhood, during my training, and throughout my career—that have in many ways shaped me as a physician, but mostly as a human being struggling to find meaning and purpose.

I recently asked my dear friend Dr. Jack Geiger—one of the world's leading public health activists—if he recalled any instances from his childhood that could have influenced his perspectives as he grew and developed. Just shy of his ninety-first birthday when we spoke about this, Jack responded immediately, recalling an incident that occurred when he was five years old. Walking with his mother on Manhattan's West Side, he encountered a man selling apples from a pushcart. Jack asked why he was doing that, and his mother gave him a five-year-old's version of the Great Depression, talking about the many people who had lost their jobs and had to do whatever they could to make sure they had food for their families.

Jack asked his mom to buy some apples; she refused, saying they didn't need apples. Jack, distraught, said, "We have to do something." Breaking away from his mother's hand, Jack ran over to the apple seller, pulled a nickel out his handkerchief, and gave it to the man, explaining that was all he had.

That's what stayed with Jack for the next eighty-six years: something is not right, *I need to fix it.* That's the story of Jack's life and, as far as I can tell, mine too.

I am determined to leave you feeling optimistic about the future. There is indeed much that can be done by government, parents, and any citizen who wants to understand how investing in children now will increase the chances of securing America's future resiliency and prosperity. These prescriptions will be described in the final chapters as a reminder to all of us that fighting for children is anything but a lost cause. And nothing could be more important.

The Future of Us

PART I
Kids Who Dream, Kids Who Can't

William, Paleontologist

Spring 1991

A gaunt, ten-year-old, light-skinned African American boy is sitting on the exam table in a mobile pediatric clinic in Brooklyn, New York. He barely makes a visual dent in the rather small exam room crowded with a hanging otoscope and ophthalmoscope set, an equipment table, and a chair. The kid is looking down, guarded, as I walk in. His flannel shirt is a size too big, and his jeans don't exactly fit either. The look is tattered and poor. He seems tired and is a little hunched. Something's missing, though. The kid is here by himself. Unusual.

I appreciate that I may be a bit overwhelming to him. He's a little ten-year-old; I'm a six-foot-one, forty-seven-year-old big guy with a stethoscope, an old Jerry Garcia tie, and a shirt pocket stuffed with papers and a ballpoint pen. "Hi. I'm Dr. Redlener. What's your name?"

"William."

"Glad to meet you, William."

As I have done thousands of times in my career, I try to draw him out with a little banter, doctor style. "How you doing? Anything bothering you?"

"No," he says, still staring at the blue carpeting under his feet.

There's no paperwork, no medical records available on this child. The nurse confirms, "He came without a chart." Right. No surprise there, not in this practice.

"Let's set him up," I say to the nurse, meaning let's start a medical record and get a basic assessment of his condition, as best as we can.

He's moderately underweight for his height, but otherwise his vital signs and physical exam—blood pressure, breath sounds, abdominal palpation—suggest no obvious medical problems. I keep up the small talk questions, like "So, how's school going?" and "How long have you been staying here?" I'm getting mostly one-word answers and an assortment of mildly nuanced shoulder shrugs. Typical for a boy his age. Still, I'm intrigued.

I go for the big question, the ultimate cliché to which almost all kids respond: "So, what do you want to be when you grow up?"

It's like I turned on a light switch. Almost every child responds. Maybe that's because to them the question means "I *care* about you."

Children are essentially dreamers, their play filled with fantasy and role playing, their dreams joyously formed, unencumbered by reality. Maybe William wants to be a firefighter or a cop, or maybe a superhero or a basketball star. Maybe he simply wants to be a dad. Whatever the fantasy, and however transient it is, children are able to imagine what might be—and innocent enough to be undaunted by adversity or reality-based barriers to success.

William looks at me; he makes serious eye contact for the first time since I walked into the exam room.

"A paleontologist," he responds. "That's what I want to be."

A paleontologist? I'd been working with children for more than twenty years—and never once heard any kid express this particular aspiration.

"Really," I say, not letting on that I was impressed by the specificity of his self-confident response. "Do you know what a paleontologist does?"

William nods. "He looks for dinosaurs, and that's what I want to do. I'd like to find a dinosaur skeleton one day."

"How did you learn about paleontology, William?" I ask, assuming that maybe a teacher had introduced him to the idea.

"I read about it in the newspaper," William replies. "Somebody showed it to me a while ago."

From his shirt pocket, William pulls out a yellowed, smudged clipping torn from the *New York Times* and proudly hands it over to me. It's a story about dinosaur remains being discovered in Alaska. It was published nearly a year before.

"That's pretty cool," I respond. "If you study hard, do well in school, I think you'll make it."

But it wouldn't be easy. Not for William.

I was examining him in the back of a mobile pediatric clinic, part of a Children's Health Fund (CHF) program that provides health care to homeless and other highly disadvantaged children.

The day I met William, we were parked on a rundown Brooklyn street in a neighborhood called Flatbush outside a worn brick building housing a foster shelter for abandoned children or children who had been removed from violent homes and broken families. This was William's temporary institutional home, where he struggled to sustain a normal childhood under a shroud of underlying sadness and a future filled with uncertainty.

A block or two east of us was Brooklyn House of Detention, one of the city's largest jails. Up and down the street were rundown buildings, insurance agencies, a few gas stations, bodegas, barbershops, and small shops. People lived in decrepit apartment buildings and in walk-ups above the stores. This was a racially and ethnically mixed neighborhood, with oppressive urban poverty being the common denominator.

William was born and raised in poverty, mostly disconnected from his biological family, on his way to becoming one of those children who would float through "the system," from one shelter to the next, maybe an occasional group home. If he was "lucky," he'd score an occasional stay with a family outside the city. In the end, William would likely age out of the system, meaning he'd turn eighteen and be out on the street. If there was to be a reasonable opportunity for him to escape the realities he had lived with since the day he was born, he would need support and guidance. He'd need people who believed in him and encouraged him to keep going.

If—and this is a big "if"—he got the support he needed, it's possible that William's dream would be realized. Maybe he'd beat the odds and somehow make it through an unsupportive, often menacing system that chewed up the aspirations of kids unfortunate enough to have been born to dysfunctional families in the squalor of sullen, poverty-stricken neighborhoods.

I shake the boy's hand and put my arm around his shoulder. I know that a ten-year-old homeless boy, without resources or a supportive family, would face extraordinary challenges slogging through a life defined by roadblocks at every turn.

Maybe the sheer incongruity of an impoverished child who harbored such a beautiful aspiration made William so unforgettable to me. Or perhaps it was just a powerful reminder of possibility and hope that can flourish in any child.

William wanted to be a dinosaur hunter, a guy who would solve some of life's big mysteries. Maybe, with a few breaks, William would one day actually find an intact *Tyrannosaurus rex* skeleton in a yet undiscovered sandpit somewhere. The prospect of a happy conclusion to William's life narrative would be highly unlikely.

It gnaws at me to admit this, but I have no idea what actually became of him. Like so many other poor, disconnected children,

I suspect that he would likely be lost in a byzantine bureaucracy of city agencies, shuttled from facility to facility, perhaps in a series of foster homes, some caring and supportive, others not so much.

Although I lost track of William's whereabouts, he was never far from mind. In the summer of 2016, some twenty-five years after we met on the mobile clinic in Brooklyn, I related William's story to an old friend and colleague, Billy Shore, founder of one of the nation's leading anti–child hunger organizations, Share Our Strength. He said nothing as I spoke, and when I finished speaking, he was still just staring at me.

"What?" I said. "Why the look?"

"Just this," Billy said. "Last year our nine-year-old, Nate, said he was interested in dinosaurs. In fact, we've taken him to the museum a number of time to see dinosaur skeletons. He has many books geared for his age on the subject, and he just loves to read about them."

"Well, that's great."

"There's more," my friend continued. "Last year my wife did some research and learned that a world-famous paleontologist, Alex Downs, was working at the Ghost Ranch in New Mexico, one of the top ten dinosaur fossil fields in the world. We contacted Professor Downs, told him about our own budding dinosaur-hunting kid, and he immediately invited us out to visit."

Billy continued, "And because we could, the three of us flew out to visit the scientist where he worked. He couldn't have been more gracious and attentive to our son, spending hours with Nate showing him some of his discoveries and stoking his budding interest in the field. It was just extraordinary. I really think the visit potentially cemented our son's interest, and I wouldn't be surprised if he actually stuck with the trajectory and ended up in research paleontology."

Now neither of us needed to say anything. It was clear that the gap between what William could possibly achieve and what my friend's boy could expect as a pathway—if he persisted in hot pursuit of an aspirational dream—could not have been wider. Possible and smooth sailing for the child of means; foreboding and essentially out of reach for William.

Clarence, Adrift

Summer 1994

It was a muggy late-summer morning, and one of the Children's Health Fund's mobile medical units was parked in front of a nondescript brick building in upper Manhattan. The street wasn't bustling by New York City standards, but people were out, some hanging out on stoops, some in front of the bodegas, playing music, talking intently to their pals and randomly to passersby. Women were pushing strollers or wheeled baskets filled with groceries. Some older dark-skinned Hispanic men, dressed in wrinkled suits, were heading to an Evangelical church on the north corner of the block.

The old brick building was a weekly destination for our mobile pediatric clinic and for the medical team which, at that point, I had led for nearly seven years. Our programs were created to bring medical care to some of the city's most indigent and underserved children. As such, we were caring for many of the children living in the city's homeless family shelter system.

By the mid-1980s the problem of homelessness had evolved from a relatively minor but sad and vexing issue, involving predominantly single adults with mental health or substance abuse issues, to a major social and economic crisis. The number of homeless people spiked to 600,000 by the end of Ronald Reagan's presidency.[1] But the big change by 1986 was the sharp rise in the number of families, as opposed to singles, who were now seeking shelter.[2] Reagan-era policies had shut down many psychiatric hospitals around the country.[3] Their services were supposed to be replaced by an aggressive proliferation of outpatient mental health clinics, but that never happened. In any case, that was not really behind the significant uptick of homeless children in cities like New York. Other forces were driving the crisis for poor families. Jobs were hard to find, especially for African Americans, whose unemployment rate was 2.77 times higher than for whites.[4] Also during this period, federal support for low-income residential housing construction waned, and there was a concurrent rise in rental rates in the inner cities. Families became homeless for any number of reasons: after fires destroyed their apartments, or because they couldn't afford the skyrocketing rents, or because they lost their jobs, or to escape domestic violence, for example. But the main culprit was a failing economic and social safety net.

By 1986, thousands of families, including some 10,000 children, were being sheltered throughout the five boroughs under conditions little better than life on the streets.[5] For the most part, these families were placed in poorly supervised "welfare hotels," or congregate shelters that were, by design, located far from their original neighborhoods. Once in the shelter system, families struggled to fulfill basic needs like clothing, food, and finding permanent housing. Getting the children to school was often a problem, and finding appropriate health care was close to impossible for many.

And over the course of a year, in addition to the children living in shelters with their families, more than 40,000 children, many like William, the budding paleontologist, would come through the foster care system.[6] After a temporary stay in a special facility or group home, most of these children were placed with relatives in what the city called "kinship environments."

But not all of the kids were so fortunate. Several thousand children would never find permanent homes. These were kids without safe or appropriate options, children with physical handicaps or behavioral issues that made finding long-term placement virtually impossible. Such children, once called "nomads" by former New York City mayor David Dinkins, spent their entire childhood going from one shelter to another—from six-bed group homes to residential facilities, from shelters in the city to placements outside the community altogether. Finally, at age eighteen, they were considered discharged from the system. In essence they "aged out," adrift on the city's streets.

So it was that summer of 1994 when we were in the mobile clinic, seeing patients from a large shelter for foster kids. As usual, I braced myself for a busy day. There were many children to be seen, mostly between six and fourteen years old. Every one of them was a story of struggle and sadness. They were from broken families, extreme poverty, their parents gone or disabled. They had struggled under conditions of overwhelming adversity, the likes of which were essentially incomprehensible to most of our medical team. More than a few had lost parents to HIV/AIDS. Some of the children were infected themselves.

At some point in the mid-morning, the facility staff brought Clarence, a twelve-year-old African American boy, into the mobile clinic. I greeted the tall, lanky child and shook his hand, asking the worker what the problem was.

"He's slow," the man stage-whispered, "and he's in a special class—and a real behavioral problem."

I asked for previous medical records and for any more information they might have on Clarence's medical or family history. Not surprisingly, very little was available—virtually nothing about family background.

We slipped into one of the small exam rooms on the unit. I tried to engage Clarence in small talk; he responded by smiling, wordlessly. His shirt clung tightly to his chest, and his pants hung loosely, a mismatched outfit obviously salvaged from the shelter's donated clothing. But when he finally spoke, he was virtually incomprehensible. I asked Clarence to sit up on the exam table. When I examined his mouth and throat, I gasped. This boy had essentially no palate. I could see into his nasal cavities through his mouth—the roof was missing entirely. This is a well-known condition called cleft palate—in Clarence's case, a complete cleft palate.

I stood there for a moment. Clarence, still smiling and sweet, was looking at me. He fidgeted, crinkling the paper that covered the exam table. I asked the nurse to take a look in the child's mouth. Neither of us could believe it. A twelve-year-old with an untreated cleft palate was unheard of in a modern, developed society. Typically, the condition is recognized at birth and treated surgically starting around four months of age. The consequences of not closing the palate include, among other things, severe delays and impairment of speech. From there, a language-impaired child from an impoverished home in a broken educational system gets labeled. He's considered severely speech delayed, erroneously considered mentally slow, and placed accordingly in school.

Socially, such children may be shunned or ridiculed by peers. Many of these children will develop secondary emotional or behavioral problems, exacerbating an already difficult situation in the classroom. By twelve, the original problems and all of the secondary consequences of a missed medical condition may have already resulted in irreversible problems. What's painful is that this social and psychological catastrophe may well have been averted by early diagnosis, appropriate care, and a supportive social system. Clarence had none of this.

Over the ensuing weeks, after a lot of digging, our team was able to produce a reasonably clear picture of Clarence's early medical history. As it turns out, he actually was diagnosed early. In his birth records the examining physician had clearly noted the absent palate. He had even recommended close monitoring and surgical follow-up. The same thing was noted repeatedly by doctors and nurses in various emergency departments that had seen Clarence for acute illnesses over the years. Young Clarence would be taken to the hospital because of high fever, for instance, and get antibiotics for an ear infection. On other occasions he'd be seen for a rash or diarrhea. Each time the doctor would note something about the palate, each time suggesting that follow-up be done.

But it never happened. Among other realities, Clarence wasn't taken to the emergency room by people who had a long-term, vested interest in him and in what might be a very complicated and expensive surgical intervention. He would be brought to the hospital for evaluation of an acute medical condition by a shelter employee or case worker "on duty." Most importantly, this boy did not have a regular source of medical care, something pediatricians refer to as a "medical home." Clarence's care took place entirely in hospital emergency departments or the occasional random clinic visit. Had he been getting regular care by a medical team that knew him and kept comprehensive medical records, the critical follow-up he needed would likely have occurred.

The fact is that Clarence's future was placed in enormous jeopardy because he lacked access to appropriate, timely health care in a setting that was committed to his long-term well-being.

At age twelve, now under the care of the Children's Health Fund teams, he finally began the treatment he should have received as an infant. That was certainly good, but much had been lost that would never be recovered.

Sadly, although we may have hoped to see vast improvements in the social adversities that led to Clarence's falling through the cracks, that hasn't been the case. In a 2016 report issued by the Children's Health Fund, data showed that more than 20 million out of some 73 million young people under the age of eighteen in the United States still lacked timely access to comprehensive health care, even though the number of children without health insurance has dropped significantly.[7]

How is this explained? It seems that many insured children face barriers of access to health care that have nothing to do with health insurance. These are children who live with their families in severe doctor-shortage communities or places where affordable transportation to get to a doctor is not available.

As for homelessness, many cities have experienced worrisome growth in the number of homeless families and children. In New York City, for instance, the average nightly shelter census of homeless children rose from about 10,000 in 1986 to nearly 24,000 three decades later.[8] In other words, more than twenty years after we first met Clarence, it was still possible to have children fall through the cracks of a health care system that simply does not work for millions of vulnerable children.

Thomas and Robert: Emergence!

Spring 1998

I've seen my share of children who successfully emerge from serious adversity—and certainly their stories are inevitably inspiring. The problem is that these are exceptional outcomes representing a very small minority of children who have the misfortune of growing up in extreme generational poverty. These are children whose parents and grandparents were poor and, if statistics are predictive, whose next generation of children will remain mired in poverty as well.

Still, it is important to recognize that adversity—even severe and prolonged adversity—does not inevitably determine outcome. Success in spite of (or sometimes because of) coping with huge challenges happens, and that has always been true. Out of war, famine, major disasters, incarceration, discrimination, psychological turmoil, and abuse of all kinds come inspiring examples of emergence. Some individuals who are personally—perhaps even genetically—resilient, gritty, and maybe lucky enough to have somebody who cared about their surviving and thriving can manage to find a pathway to a successful life. Sometimes we recognize them and may call them heroes. Sometimes they thrive, perfectly content, in obscurity.

Thomas was twelve and his brother Robert nine when his father lost his job in Kingston, Jamaica, putting himself and the two boys in a precarious economic situation, starting with an eviction notice from their modest one-bedroom apartment. Dad and the boys' mother had separated a year prior, and she was living in a small spare bedroom of a relative in the Bronx. Her departure had been traumatic for the brothers, and the latest seemingly irresolvable family financial crisis greatly exacerbated the level of stress and anxiety that the family was experiencing. Robert was acting out in school, grades dropping and reports to the principal rising. Thomas refused to go to school at all. Their unemployed father was beside himself, increasingly depressed, unable to manage the boys' issues while focused on trying to find work. In desperation, a decision was made to send the brothers to New York City in hopes that their mother would care for them, at least until their dad could get his situation stabilized.

This turned out to be more wishful thinking than a viable plan. Not only was their mother living under circumstances that could not accommodate the boys, but when they arrived in New York, they learned that their mother was four months pregnant. Within a week of their arrival, the brothers were placed in the city's foster care system, assigned to a series of small group home settings. And that's where I found them.

Thomas was brought to me for a check-up.

"Thomas, I'm Dr. Redlener, and I want to speak with you for a few minutes, do a quick exam, and make sure that you're healthy. How are you doing?" The boy looked down and said nothing.

"OK if I ask you a few questions?" That at least got a quick shoulder shrug. But clearly this was going to be a challenging conversation. I asked the nurse to push back my next appointment to accommodate what I suspected would be a difficult conversation. Indeed, Thomas had a good deal on his mind, and eventually, bit by bit, over what turned out to be many visits over a six-month period, the story emerged. Besides the details about what

14

his family was going through, it was clear that the young man was deeply worried, not so much about himself but about his brother, who was with him in the group home, about his pregnant mother, and about his father in Jamaica—all of it seemingly on his twelve-year-old shoulders.

Eventually, Thomas and I bonded, and he learned to trust me. We did what we could to address the multiple issues he was worried about, starting with getting his asthma under control. It is worth noting that dealing effectively with this medical issue was straightforward, by the book, and rapidly resolved. But the family challenges, the stress, the academic continuity both boys needed—that's where the care and support of these boys got really tough.

So, what exactly was my role as a physician? Did it stop with my writing prescriptions for his asthma medications? Hardly. The circumstances that actually influenced Thomas's well-being were not predominantly medical, not covered in my old textbooks or in the scores of lectures I heard in med school and throughout my training. This situation, like so many that involve children living with multiple adversities, is about health and well-being defined in the broadest sense of those concepts. Doctors need to be sufficiently aware of the entire range of issues affecting their patients, the children who are under their care.

Thomas and Robert got the full range of comprehensive services from the Children's Health Fund: medical care, case management, psychological counseling, academic support, career advice, and so on. We stayed with these kids as their mom gave birth to their new little sister, as their dad came to New York and found a decent job, and as they got their act together and graduated from high school. We were "there" when the family reunited and moved into a good apartment, finally.

It should be noted that before the boys were bought into the Children's Health Fund's network of care, they were getting, at best, random health care for check-ups and a trip to the closest emergency room if they had an acute medical problem. They needed much more. CHF was able to provide substantial attention to the health, psychological, and social issues that were standing in the way of their successful adaptation to their adopted country, the pressures of being in the foster care system, and the academic challenges in their new schools.

Robert went to a community college and landed a great job as a building superintendent. Thomas was accepted to and graduated from a prestigious New York college and went on to finish a nursing program, as well as a master's degree in social work. As of 2015, he had successfully ventured into writing and publishing children's books.

Success stories—hard to come by in my work, but always appreciated, always reminding us that almost every child has potential and that success can, indeed, prevail over adversity. But it doesn't happen on its own. The commitment of supporting adults, the availability of decent schools, and robust social support systems all make a difference.

So, how much credit does the doctor get for a successful child who emerges from a tough environment and actually makes good? That's not clear, but humility is in order here because many factors will influence the trajectory of a child, including his or her personality, grit, and the presence of a caring adult.

That caring adult, first of all, must believe that almost anything is possible for the child who is under his or her protective wing. Second, that adult must be committed to doing whatever can be done to mitigate and buffer the conditions that would otherwise blunt aspirations and turn off the dream machine essential to any successful childhood. This assumption of responsibility for protecting a child from the firestorms of a dangerous childhood may be taken consciously by a parent, a physician, a social worker, or any adult in the child's orbit.

The point is to realize that whoever assumes that role is vital to a child's ability to escape adversity by serving as a protective buffer for a child awash in challenges, providing consistent support, positive reinforcement, and a reminder that the dreams of childhood can, one day, materialize.

LaTisha, Marine Biologist

Fall 2014

It's a chilly early November, and I'm sitting in the crowded waiting room of the CHF's South Bronx Center for Child Health and Resiliency. I had come up to the center for a late afternoon meeting with the clinic's senior staff, including my wife, Karen, then executive director of Montefiore Medical Center's community pediatrics program. The agenda was to be a discussion about an upcoming site visit by a major donor looking to get a feel for what exactly we did up here in the South Bronx, a community often considered an urban no-man's-land by the wealthy Wall Streeter whose usual habitat was Manhattan's Upper East Side.

We had designed and built the nearly four-year-old health center to be a welcoming and efficiently functioning medical destination for children and their families. A round, sweeping low-rise counter staffed by friendly, smiling registrars was the first thing families saw when they entered the facility. The décor was all about soothing, coordinated pastels; the walls were covered with unique, child-friendly art and bright accent panels.

As I sit in the waiting room, filled with the bustle and buzz of babies, children, and their parents, I'm not thinking about anything particularly profound—just a little zoned out after a long day. To my right are a few couples with an assortment of kids and some young moms tenderly holding babies or reading to toddlers on their laps. Directly across from me, a dad sits smiling at his young child, who is playing with a stuffed animal. Sitting next to him is a teenager, ball cap askew, baggy pants, a Beats headset

17

attached to his phone, eyes lightly closed, and a hoodie—classic adolescent chic for this part of the city.

There's a young African American girl who catches my eye. She's adorable, looks about nine or ten, and she's holding a couple of small toy fish—or that's what they seem to be. I get up and wander over.

"Nice fish," I say.

"Well, this one is actually a barracuda," she says, holding a green plastic toy in her left hand. "And this other one is a tiger shark," she adds, showing me the other little model.

"Oh yeah," I respond. "I couldn't really see them from where I was sitting. Are they the man-eating variety?"

"Well, not the barracuda," she says assertively, "But you gotta watch out for the shark. Those tigers attack people swimming in the ocean and eat just about anything."

"Wow! That sounds scary."

"Yeah. But not as scary as the great whites. Those suckers attack people all the time and they're huge."

"Thanks for that. I will definitely try to stay out of their way. By the way, what's your favorite kind of shark?"

"Me? I like the hammerheads. They look really weird. Ever see one?"

"No. But how do you so much about sharks?"

"From my teacher. She told us about this book. I borrowed it from school—and then my mom got me a video all about sharks."

"Pretty good. Listen, I'm just curious, what grade are you in?"

"I'm in fourth. My school's just a few blocks from here."

"So, who brought you here today?"

"My worker," the child says matter-of-factly, pointing to a middle-aged woman sitting on the other side of the waiting room.

"Mind if I say hello to her?" I ask.

"No. And my name is LaTisha. What's yours?"

"I'm Irwin. And by the way, young LaTisha, what do you want to be when you grow up?"

Without a minute of hesitation, this beautiful, engaging, adorable kid who lives and goes to school in one of the most troubled urban communities in America looks up at me and says, with unabashed conviction and clarity, "Well, I'm going to be a marine biologist."

"I'm not surprised," I say. "Sounds like a great idea."

I approach her "worker," who identifies herself as Gail. Just to establish my credibility, I let her know that I'm the pediatrician who founded the Children's Health Fund. She's pleasant enough, and we engage in a little small talk. She doesn't say, and I don't ask, why LaTisha is here with her—not her Mom—but she is clearly very familiar with this family.

"So, why is LaTisha here today?" I ask.

"It's her asthma. Mom said she was up all night coughing and was too tired to go to school this morning. She finally perked up, I'm happy to see."

We talk for a few minutes about LaTisha's very impressive knowledge about sharks. Gail tells me that the kid is really into the subject, and her mother is very encouraging. I ask if LaTisha's ever been to an aquarium.

"Almost. A few months ago LaTisha's mom and a couple of other parents in their building found a way to organize a trip. But when they got there, the place was closed. It was pretty sad," says Gail.

"I'll say. Think they'll reschedule?

"Doubt it. It cost them a lot to get there, and times are pretty tough now."

I don't respond.

Gail continues: "That girl is hangin' in there. But her family is pretty messed up. Her father is in prison, and her younger brother is in a kinship foster home. Worst of all, Mom has a serious addiction issue. And they never have enough food stamps left at the end of the month." She pauses and looks away. "I'm not really supposed to, but I try to bring them some groceries when I visit."

I get the picture. The fact that LaTisha's sole available parent, her mother, is an addict doesn't bode well for this child with big, lofty aspirations. To begin with, studies have shown that children raised by drug addicts are significantly prone to developing emotional, social, and behavioral adjustment problems. Children of substance-abusing parents are more than twice as likely as their peers to develop a substance-abuse problem of their own.[9] Many of these children demonstrate psychological or behavioral problems. And all of these issues can adversely affect school performance. In other words, young LaTisha is at high risk for never being able to realize her own very precious dreams.

I look up at a picture on the waiting room wall. It's a globe with some smiling children. It says, "The World Is Waiting—Let's Go!"

I look over at LaTisha, who's playing with her toy sharks, moving them through the air as if they were riding the ocean waves.

I am thinking that this is a kid who *needs* to become a marine biologist. For her sake, of course, and also for the world waiting for her to take her place in a society that desperately needs every child to be a success story, to realize aspirations that will lead to a productive, fulfilled life, not slip back into the terrible cycle of poverty and failure that, generation after generation, consumes families like LaTisha's.

And here I am contemplating all of this in the waiting room of a South Bronx clinic where I met a charming nine-year-old enjoying a short respite from the streets and the stress she has lived with since the day she was born.

Raymond, Graphic Designer

Winter 2015

It's a bitterly cold mid-January afternoon. I am in the St. John's Place Family Shelter in Brooklyn, this time in the impoverished

Crown Heights community, a neighborhood once notorious for civil unrest involving violent conflicts between the African American and Jewish communities. This shelter was opened in 1990 by New York's Settlement Housing Fund expressly to provide a civilized option for homeless families who would otherwise find themselves forced into one of the squalid congregate shelters or welfare hotels that proliferated in the city.[10]

In essence, the unrelenting problem of homelessness among families that prompted us in 1987 to create the Children's Health Fund, a special comprehensive health services for children in the shelters, had persisted and, sadly, grown substantially by the time I met Raymond in 2015. Unlike Clarence, Raymond was never in the foster system, but his childhood was spent living in extreme economic fragility, housing instability, and long stays in shelters in the metropolitan area.

Estimates suggest that from the mid-1980s through 2016, the number of homeless New York City families increased from approximately 4,000 to more than 14,000. That meant that in the late 1980s, some 10,000 children lived in New York City shelters on any given night, and by 2016 that count had more than doubled to nearly 24,000 children as an average nightly census.[11] Even with the help of hardworking city government agencies, newly homeless families simply could not find affordable housing in a city that was otherwise thriving economically and on a mad dash toward maximum gentrification. That left thousands of homeless families with little choice other than "single-room occupancy" (SRO) and decrepit welfare hotels whose owners were repeatedly cited for violating health and housing standards; many of the buildings urgently needed repair for everything from nonworking plumbing, broken elevators, and peeling paint to vermin infestations and broken room locks.

Most of these facilities could have and should have been torn down to make room for new construction of apartment buildings or small business venues. But the city urgently needed a place to warehouse thousands of homeless singles and families who had little likelihood of finding affordable permanent housing. With a combination of funds from the city and the federal government, private owners of these emergency shelters kept these decrepit facilities intact. In effect, they were a virtual gold mine for the owners, who exploited the city's desperation—and the availability of emergency shelter dollars—charging from $1,500 to sometimes as much as $3,000 per room per month to "house" a homeless family. And it was full occupancy 365 days a year! But New York City was committed to finding shelter for the homeless, even if more than $100 million would eventually be spent to keep people, including families and children, off the streets.

Hearing statistics about homelessness is not enough to appreciate the actual impact on the families caught up in the destructive morass of prolonged displacement under highly adverse conditions. One of the mass shelters housed up to a thousand people, including families with kids and homeless singles with drug, alcohol, and criminal histories, for periods that averaged eighteen months or more.

Think about that. Terrified, poor, and out of options, single parents with babies, toddlers, and school-age children in tow would be spending more than a year in shelters intermingled with adult drug addicts and people with serious mental health problems.

And in the privately owned welfare hotels, a common bathroom could be shared by many people, some of whom might be prostitutes or drug dealers. Access to school, hot meals, or health care for children was severely impaired. To this day, no one has been able to fully measure the long-term effects of homelessness on many of the children who lived through these very tough years. That is not to say that none of the children enduring these conditions got through unscathed. In fact, many kids proved to be surprisingly resilient to the stress around them, often buffered by a strong parent or other adult figure who was able to protect them from the ubiquitous psychological and sometimes physical trauma of urban homelessness.

But in general, for the majority of children trapped in the shelters and the welfare hotels, childhood was a living hell.

By 2000, the small nugget of good news in the "management" of homeless families was the elimination of placements in the large, dehumanizing congregate shelters and the so-called welfare hotels that had been so prevalent in the late 1980s and early 1990s. These worst of the worst shelters were in part replaced by so-called Tier II shelters, some of which provide clean facilities, a working kitchen, and a private bathroom. Unfortunately, with the recent dramatic growth of the homeless population, many families with children continue to be placed in terrible public housing facilities in some of the city's most treacherous neighborhoods.

That said, St. John's Place, and other facilities like it, were expressly designed as antidotes to the welfare hotels. St. John's provides clean, furnished apartments with private baths and kitchens in a secure building. It isn't fancy by any stretch, but it is a relatively safe place for children. A flourishing garden tended by the residents provides fresh vegetables and a source of pride.

Raymond, a sweet-faced fifteen-year-old boy, born some four years after we started Children's Health Fund in 1987, sits down across from me at a table in the shelter director's office, staring anxiously at the floor. This young man is part of the latest generation of lost and struggling kids, and I am still waiting for some kind of revolution, a wake-up call that would lead to the elimination of homelessness and poverty that is still grinding down the dreams of more than 16 million children in America.

There is no eye contact for the first minutes of our conversation. Raymond is clearly small for his age; his pant legs are bunched up at his ankles, and the sleeves of his zippered fleece flap loosely on his arms. But what strikes me is the huge shoulder bag—worn, stained, strapped across the boy's chest, jammed full of what, I have no idea.

I greet Raymond and introduce myself. He nods, eyes fixed on the empty table.

Raymond unstraps the shoulder bag from his chest and clutches it in his arms. I ask him a few questions. "How long have you been living in the shelter? Where do you go to school? Who lives with you?" His replies are polite, but soft, almost muted. He says, "About five weeks" and "In Brooklyn" and "I live with my mom and stepfather. And my sister." Still no eye contact.

I explain that I want to talk about his life and his future. Raymond glances at his bag.

"What's in there?" I ask. "I'm dying of curiosity."

Like William, the boy who aspired to be a paleontologist, Raymond suddenly raises his head and looks right at me, with a big smile spread across his face. He actually startles me.

"It's my art work," he says. "I always have it with me."

"I'd love to see your work, if I may."

From the worn, dirty shoulder bag, Raymond pulls out dozens of portfolio books, carefully spreading them on the table.

What I see is dazzling. On page after page, in book after book, are hundreds of stunning images of characters, still-life drawings of fruit and flowers, science fiction–like industrial designs, logos he has created for real or imagined companies or products, sketches of people and scenes. There is a beautiful pencil drawing of an art teacher who inspired and encouraged him, even as a fourth grader. Raymond clearly has tremendous talent.

There is no stopping him now. Words tumble out. Raymond explains that he first became interested in drawing when he was seven, and he has saved every piece of artwork since then.

"See this?" he says, opening one book. "I think this was the first drawing I ever did." He points out an exquisitely detailed pencil drawing of a cartoon character. Then his fingers move to a drawing on the opposite page. "And here," he says, "is an updated version I did last year."

It's a beautiful color rendition of the same image, more sophisticated and clearly done with a far more mature technique.

After going through almost everything, he says, "Hey, do you want to see some of my computer-designed work?"

"Hell, yes!" I reply.

Raymond pulls a flash drive out his pocket and grins. "It's all here. I'll email it to you."

"Great," I respond. "You have a computer?"

He shakes his head, grin fading. "I do. But it's old and not really working. I try to use the computer room at school."

"Raymond," I say, leaning toward him. "Your work is just beautiful. Tell me what you want to do after you graduate from high school."

"I want to go to art school and learn graphic design," he says immediately, his brown eyes once again fixed down at the table. "I would be so happy if I could do that for the rest of my life."

No doubt, I think. "Can you make this happen?"

"Sure," he says, beginning to put his work back into his bag. "Why not?"

"Of course you will," I say with as much assurance as I can muster. But I know better.

As with many precariously situated families, Raymond's family's fall into homelessness had been steep, fast, and persistent. Years earlier, the family was doing okay, with income sufficient for just making ends meet. Then his stepdad was injured on the job, and it was downhill from there. They ended up in the shelter system and, as with so many others, breaking out was not so easy.

Because his living situation, essentially shelter to shelter, was always changing, the shy teenager avoided making friends, rarely speaking with classmates. Everything was always in flux, but he found peace and stability in his artwork. And with tremendous effort, he managed to pass all of his courses, regularly winning praise from teachers for his wonderful drawings.

Through some inexplicable force of will, Raymond's parents were still chasing the dream of a better life, somewhere. Anywhere.

But in the middle of a tough Northeast winter, they ended up in a homeless shelter deep in the heart of Brooklyn.

Raymond and his sister have asthma. This is the most prevalent pediatric chronic illness, being diagnosed in 8.6 percent of all children,[12] and found in an astounding 33 percent of homeless children in New York City.[13] In any case, recurrent wheezing and poorly controlled asthma were taking a toll on Raymond and his family. They usually, but not always, had medicine and inhaler pumps to treat the symptoms when it was just too difficult to breathe or impossible to sleep through the coughing spasms. Like many other homeless kids, they had the prescriptions for their breathing meds written in crowded, dingy exam rooms of the public hospital closest to whatever shelter they happened to be in.

I couldn't know for sure, but it is likely that some combination of changing weather, the stress of constant displacement from one shelter to another, and his parents struggling to sustain some semblance of a normal life triggered the asthma attacks. And as they became increasingly frequent, he missed many days of school.

Raymond also tells me he has "some kind of eye problem."

"Like what, exactly?"

"Sometimes, when I'm reading, my vision gets blurry and I can't see the letters," he explains.

"What do you do? Have you seen a doctor for this?"

"Not really," Raymond says. "I usually just blink a few times and it seems to get better."

I make a mental note and the next day arrange for him to see one of the eye doctors who work with our primary care teams.

The family has been living in St. John's for just a few weeks. The director has big plans for more improvements, including a computer room. But it isn't there yet, and Raymond has only his shoulder bag to carry his personal art gallery, his life story, and the dreams he is determined to hang onto despite unforeseeable challenges.

I stare at Raymond, trying to absorb what he has said, the whole of it—the love of art, the traumas, the uncontrolled asthma, the deprivations, and, especially, the extraordinary barriers that stand between him and a fulfilled life, free of poverty, working at a job he would love.

The painful reality is that millions of children like William, LaTisha, and Raymond struggle in small towns, cities, and rural areas across America—impoverished children with the richest of dreams, many with talents and inexplicable perseverance who may or may not overcome the conditions over which they have no control. Many of these kids are brilliant or artistic, many filled with undaunted dynamism. They could be our next generation of statesmen, generals, physicists, entrepreneurs, doctors, artists, scientists, and teachers.

They are neither less than nor different from middle- or upper-class children when it comes to their desire to live a full and successful life. This recurrent story, the impact of enduring poverty, is about the rise and fall of aspirations extinguished by adversities that most Americans can barely imagine.

I pull out of my thoughts and ask, "Raymond, what do you think might stop you from realizing your dreams?"

He looks at me for a moment. I think he may cry—or maybe that's me I'm thinking about. He looks suddenly older than his fifteen years.

"We have to move too much. We have no money, and I know my family won't be able to buy me the books I'll need. I have some art supplies now, but I worry that they'll be gone soon because I draw so much."

He pulls a small tin of colored drawing pencils from his bag, many of them just stubs. "My teacher gave me these."

"Raymond, clearly you love art—and you're damned good at it. I think your dreams *will* come true if you stick with it."

I try to sound like I mean it. I can't tell if he believes me.

Is there some way—any way—I can help this impoverished homeless kid with big aspirations?

"Raymond, have you been to any of the art museums in New York?"

"No, sir," he responds. "I've never been to any museum. Never in my life."

"Never?"

He shook his head.

I think about this minor travesty as we leave the office. I see Luis, the shelter director, in an adjacent waiting room, so I ask Raymond to hang back for a minute.

"Luis, this kid is a wonderful artist and could have a great career ahead of him—*if* he can break out of the cycle of poverty his family is in." Luis sighs and shrugs. He is a wonderful shelter director in an awful system, and he can only do so much.

"This boy has never been to a museum," I tell him.

Luis grimaces. "I don't know what will happen to families like his," he says. "I have no magic answer to solve the poverty issue." Then a flicker of a smile comes across his face. "But the museum situation I can deal with."

He gets an idea. "I'll organize a van trip to the Museum of Modern Art for Raymond and some of the other teens staying here." Now we're talking. Within a few weeks, a bunch of teenagers who had been living their lives disconnected from the cornucopia of art and culture in their own city got to see one of the world's great museums. For some, those few hours of invested time, a rented bus, a light lunch, and an unforgettable experience would help solidify a sense of belonging in society and offer up what could be a bit of hope that, somehow or other, it would be okay to imagine a future that would be fulfilling and meaningful.

By March of 2016, Raymond and his family were living in Camden, a dingy impoverished South New Jersey urban wasteland. "Why there?" I asked when he told me that the family was planning on moving. He explained that they were sick of living in shelters and they had heard that apartments were very affordable. Plus they had lived there some years prior.

"But, Raymond, what about school?" I asked. "You're doing well in Brooklyn, and you have a lot of support for your artwork."

"I think it will be fine. Anyway, I have no choice," said Raymond. I didn't say it, but I thought, "You've got that right."

That's the problem right there. For so many children and their families who are stuck in the groove and grip of poverty, choices are limited for everything—where they live, what they can purchase, the capacity to make education decisions that lead them to the lives to which they aspire, the ability to visit a museum or travel someplace just for the adventure of it, the clothes they want, the privacy we all crave sometimes, the ability to save for the future, the resources to choose healthy food, the money to pay for a blazer that Raymond needed to go with his class on a field trip to a New York art gallery that was to show his work or buy a uniform for the baseball team, the capacity to once in a damn blue moon to eat in a restaurant with tablecloths, the big and small things of life, the non-extravagant things and possibilities that should be accessible for any American kid. Those are the choices that I have, that my children and grandchildren benefit from, that should be Raymond's American birthright, too.

Raymond called from Camden one Saturday morning in late March. He was coughing and hard to understand, but he told me that he had been sick for four or five days with high fevers, cough, and wheezing. He was feeling generally lousy. He told me that his mom had taken him to an emergency room at Cooper Hospital in Camden a couple of days before, but his symptoms just were getting worse.

"What did they do for you, Ray?"

"Not much. Just told me to stay home from school and take Motrin and Tylenol."

"No blood tests? No x-rays?" I asked. "What about any prescriptions?"

"No, nothing like that."

I told Raymond to go back to the emergency room now and have them reevaluate the situation. They'd need to carefully reexamine him, order the right tests, make a more informed diagnosis, and treat accordingly. He agreed to go. I asked him to call me back when he was in the ER so he could hand the phone to the doctor who's treating him. The well-reputed hospital was affiliated with a new and innovative medical school, part of Rowan University, and I was at least comfortable that he was likely to get good care.

More than an hour later, Raymond called back.

"Where are you?" I asked.

"We're heading back home," Raymond said through the coughing. "The bus never showed up, and my mom doesn't have money for a cab. We'll ask my stepdad if he can help me out." Fine, I said, just keep me posted—my plan being to prepay a car service by credit card to pick him up at his apartment building and take him to the hospital.

Eventually the story ended okay. He got to the hospital by car service, and he was evaluated properly. The treating physician told me that the chest x-ray looked clear and his blood count was not suggestive of a bacterial infection that might have required antibiotics, so a presumptive diagnosis of influenza was made. Because Raymond and his doctors felt that his asthma was under control, just symptomatic treatment was recommended to manage his viral flu, in addition to keeping up with his asthma attack prevention medications.

But here's the problem that is a grave issue for millions of children. There may well be a perfectly fine hospital or clinic that would see a family like Raymond's on Medicaid, the government's health insurance program for the poor—or, if necessary, provide care at no charge or at a reduced rate according to the family's income. But for an economically stressed family, just getting to the doctor or hospital is the challenge. Raymond's family didn't have a car. And although there was an affordable metro bus system, service was generally minimal and essentially skeletal on the weekends.

According to the 2016 Distressed Communities Index published by the Economic Innovation Group, Camden, New Jersey, was rated the most distressed city in the United States. Average family income there is 36.4 percent of New Jersey's overall average. Nearly a third of the population has not graduated from high school.[14] With the city's tax base in a permanent slump, Camden had to pare down all government services, including public transportation—that in itself being a health care issue and an example of the realities of living poor in America.

Asthma is the most common chronic illness among children of all socioeconomic groups. But the challenges and consequences faced by poor children with the disease versus how the condition plays out for children whose families are not economically stressed is striking—and informative.

This is how it goes for children with asthma who have timely access to decent medical care: Typically, a child with, say, persistent cough and wheezing is evaluated by a doctor, a diagnosis is made, and medications are prescribed both to prevent acute asthma flare-ups and to treat an attack if there is a breakthrough. The health care team provides asthma management education, teaching families about factors that could trigger acute flare-ups and how to avoid or manage them. If the medications are correct and the family sufficiently educated about controlling the disease, emergency room visits or hospitalizations are rarely necessary.

But the realities of asthma management for a child living in poverty are strikingly different—and far more dangerous. If there is not regular access to a "medical home," opportunities for early diagnosis, proper prescriptions, and asthma education are severely limited. The medical care of childhood asthma under such circumstances becomes a series of emergency runs to the nearest hospital, often so late in the course of an attack that treatment must be done in an inpatient setting, occasionally in the pediatric intensive care unit, where a breathing tube and mechanical ventilator may be necessary.

But the outcomes of poorly controlled asthma go far beyond a child's medical well-being. There are other important consequences that can even affect a child's academic success or the family's economic security. Children with undertreated asthma often suffer from severe nighttime coughing. This commonly results in disturbed and restless sleep or even difficulty falling asleep. With school-age children, parents may keep them home. These are the children at risk for chronic absenteeism—a condition highly associated with academic failure.

Even if they go to school, children with unchecked asthma are likely to be too exhausted to concentrate in class, sometimes chastised by an unknowing teacher for failing to pay attention. That's why we call undiagnosed or undertreated asthma a "health barrier to learning." Worse still, the perceptions of teachers, parents, and even their peers get internalized by the child, creating a negative self-image that is reinforced by ongoing criticisms and mislabeling. Children start to fall behind, academic success becomes increasingly elusive, and aspirations for a productive, fulfilling future seem more and more out of reach.

And there is always the possibility of an asthma attack so severe that an ambulance must be called—a situation traumatic for the child and very disruptive to the rest of the class. I've spoken to principals of inner city elementary schools who report having to call an ambulance three or four times a month to transport a child with respiratory distress to the emergency room.

Sometimes a parent's job is at risk if he or she stays out of work to care for a sick child. At the least, a parent who stays up with a wheezing child during the night may be too exhausted to function in the workplace.

So what does this have to do with Raymond, coughing and sick, waiting in America's poorest city for a bus that never came to take him to the hospital to get the care he needed? What does Camden's barely functioning metro bus system have to do with asthma, poor children, and life success?

It starts with understanding the underpinnings of what it takes to have a robust, effective health care system that is "user-friendly" and equitable, accessible to everyone regardless of economic status, race, or geography. For decades, state-of-the-art hospitals and medical schools have been the primary focus of building a modern health care system, the citadels of advanced medical practice and technology integrated services.

However, in terms of real access to the fruits of advanced health services, and even to basic primary medical care, challenges have become intractable, leaving many Americans unable to get to a health care provider because of barriers ranging from the cost of care to maldistribution of doctors and clinics to public transportation deficiencies. These factors all matter to people living in the margins. And while the Affordable Care Act (ACA) has dramatically reduced the number of uninsured Americans, much work remains in terms of assuring actual access to health care services.

Most concerning at the time of this writing are the threats articulated by the Trump administration and the Congress, who seem determined to repeal the ACA. If the repeal efforts are successful, that would represent a remarkable step backward for many families who have finally gotten the security and comfort of having access to health care that every American should have.

Most people don't realize how many "health care deserts," or doctor-shortage communities, there are in the United States. The federal government tracks the distribution of medical professionals in the nation; if a community has less than one doctor for every 3,500 citizens, it is declared a Health Professional Shortage Area, or HPSA. The latest data, as of January 2016, show more than 6,000 federally designated HPSAs (two-thirds of them rural communities, one-third urban) in which at least 60 million Americans live, including 10–15 million children.[15]

This does not mean that everybody who lives in an HPSA doesn't get care; it just means that the very act of getting an appointment at a doctor's office is far more difficult. For the poor, especially those who experience other adversities, access to care can be overwhelmingly difficult—as it was with Raymond's tough trip to the hospital. Even though their rental house was just a few miles from the hospital, he was really stuck in terms of how to get there. The bus didn't show up, and his parents had no money.

Nationally, the Children's Health Fund has found that between 3.5 and 4 million children each year miss primary care checkups and follow-ups for chronic illnesses.[16] No bus, no subway, no affordable taxi service, no working car? In many places around the nation, this means you're out of luck if you need a doctor. You could call 911 and get an ambulance to respond, but who would call an ambulance to get to a clinic for a routine immunization, an ear infection follow-up—or an asthma management visit?

For many poor families with few resources and limited, if any, public transportation, getting routine care becomes "optional." So for children in families with multiple adversities, like poverty or homelessness, getting to the medical facility for anything that seems to be mild or routine drops far down the ladder of family priorities. Finding decent employment, looking for stable, affordable housing, and other issues may well be the most important day-to-day responsibilities. The children unlucky enough to be burdened with asthma become the ones who are most likely to live with chronic fatigue, high rates of absenteeism, and negative labeling by schools—a chain of events that often leads to poor academic performance, reduced chances of timely graduation from high school, and a highly constrained ability to imagine and realize dreams of a fulfilled life.

There is more here than just a call for logical policies based on understanding the long-term social benefit of making sure every child, regardless of economic status, gets high-quality and timely medical care. There is a compelling economic case to be made as well.

A study authored by CHF experts found that for every child with asthma properly treated in doctors' offices and clinics with evidence-proven protocols and medications, the "system" saves more than $4,000 because of reduced frequency of emergency room visits and hospitalizations.[17] With asthma seen in 8.6 percent of the general child population, rising to 33 percent among homeless children in cities like New York, we're talking serious dollars in savings generated by properly managing this illness alone.

These data might even appeal to those who don't relate to Mother Theresa's philosophy of providing good care to people in need purely as humanitarian acts of kindliness. Beyond that, there are real and practical reasons for doing the right thing in terms of the nation's future resiliency. So, maybe even for hard-core conservatives, small-government enthusiasts, and hedge funders, who always want to understand the "return on investment," even for government programs designed to assist people living in poverty, the case has been made.

Meanwhile, Raymond and his family seemed to be getting by in Camden when I last heard from him. And there was big news, too. Raymond had gotten accepted to a local branch campus of Rutgers University and would be starting classes in the fall. He was still looking to major in graphic arts, but then my young pal observed, "You never know. Maybe I'll find something else that's really interesting!"

Maybe he will, I thought. In spite of the challenges Raymond faces, in terms of persistent poverty and housing instability, he is fortunate to have an intact family, loving parents, and his own internal resiliency—precisely the kind of attributes that make me guardedly optimistic about Raymond's future.

Schools Filled with Dreamers,
Neighborhoods of Adversity

It's almost noon, and the cafeteria at P.S. 140 in the Bronx is filled with adorableness in the form of happy, beautiful, and eager children, kindergartners through third graders. The first lunch shift is over, and the room is buzzing. Children are laughing, but staying in their seats and chattering with their pals. I am watching them from the doorway, but stand aside when they are dismissed, filing out of the cafeteria, headed back to their classrooms; teachers are standing by, keeping a watchful eye on the brood.

It's impossible to take my eyes off these children—and I can't help thinking about my own children when they were this age of wonder and joy. I remember, too, as they got older and more complicated and became aware, at least unconsciously, of the real world, where it's not all possible and not always simple. Certainly every age has its joys, and we, like so many parents, loved every landmark, every accomplishment, even through the setbacks and disappointments, also inevitable realities of every childhood.

And when our own children finally reached middle school and beyond, I remember missing those early years, babies in high chairs at the diner, cutie-pie toddlers learning to play and interact with peers, testing independence from Karen and me, kindergartners and first graders, seemingly awed by their new ability to read the written word.

And for the most fortunate of my generation, there comes a second round of pure joy. It's when we become grandparents and can see these new kids in our lives. We watch them grow, unencumbered by the direct responsibilities of parenting, left only with a renewed sense of the future through the lives of the next generation.

That was my silent reverie at that school in the South Bronx, watching those kids in the cafeteria. And that was what was on my mind when I thought about how differently these children would experience life than my own children did. For sure, we had our own terrible setbacks—one of ours going through a hellish adolescence, others with very serious medical problems, from meningitis to severe infections and accidents, and the ultimate unspeakable sorrow of losing one of our gorgeous children in a terrible accident.

But no matter what we had to cope with or grieve for or adapt to, there was never a moment when we doubted the possibility of our children being able to envision a future of accomplishing *almost* anything they dreamed of.

Could six-year-old Michael Redlener, a talented Little League and, later, high school pitcher and first baseman who loved the New York Yankees, ever have a real shot at playing major league baseball? Not really. But he could dream about being a historian, majoring in the subject at a prestigious liberal arts college. And he could envision himself changing his mind, getting into medical school, and becoming a highly respected emergency medicine doctor. He did that. He could see himself married to the love of his life, a successful woman, also a doctor, and raising his own children, Naomi, Aaron, and Sam. He did that, too. And David, who became a lawyer, married Judith, and had two wonderful children, Caleb and Mia. That happened. And Stephanie, who married Arthur, brought Alia into our family, and gave birth to the irresistible Auren. All of that happened as well. What's more, the whole cluster of Redlener grandchildren will have a good shot at achieving their dreams and fulfilling the potential they were born with. That's good, of course, and I'm grateful that they'll all have the opportunities that have been brought to them on six little silver platters

And then there are the children of P.S. 140. They, too, like my own children, were laughing and dreaming, their faces filled with joy, even though the rest of the day might not go so well. More than 20 percent of these children would return to a homeless shelter after school, some having been in facility after facility for a year or more, many being raised by a single struggling parent. Some would miss school because the shelter's single washing machine was on the blink and they didn't have a spare set of clean clothes; others would be absent because their asthma was acting up and they couldn't get to the doctor, or they had severe pain from a dental cavity and Mom couldn't find a dentist that would take Medicaid, the government-issued health insurance that reimbursed so little that few practicing dentists would accept poor children as patients.

Children at P.S. 140 may have been dreaming, but their moms were struggling to find housing and secure nutritious food. College? A career? A decent job eventually? Nearly every parent of every homeless child wanted those aspirations to materialize for their children; very few could imagine how any of this could happen.

"So, Shandra," I once asked a twenty-eight-year-old mother of two children, "What do you hope for your kids?"

"Mostly, right now, that they get home safely from school," she said. "If they go down the wrong street and run into one of the dope gangs, there will be trouble. I worry about that every day. I usually try to get to school and walk them home. But when I am working—which I need to do—I can't always make it."

"Yes," I said, "it's hard to imagine carrying that fear around every day. But I was asking about 'hope' in a longer view sense. What do you think they want to be when they grow up? What do *you* hope for them?"

"I have thought about that a lot. My eleven-year-old wants to be a teacher, and I know she'll need to go to college. I just have no idea how that could ever happen." She continued, "And my nine-year-old says he wants to be a professional basketball player, and that's not going to happen. And when I ask about his second choice, he says 'a doctor.' That's because he met a wonderful doctor at the clinic last year and thinks that is something he'd really like to do. I don't think that's ever going happen, any more than him becoming a basketball player."

I thought about that conversation and so many others just like it. Dreams are dreamt, for sure, but they are wispy and unrealizable for many children who are living outside the margins of what we call the mainstream. And there are millions of children for whom the basic capacity to dream is there, but the ability to get from here to there is well out of reach.

P.S. 140 is one of three very low performing elementary schools in New York City that the CHF has identified as a Healthy and Ready to Learn Pilot School. There's another pilot school in the South Bronx, and a third in Harlem. In two of the schools, fewer than 10 percent of the third graders can read at grade level.

The CHF teams work in the schools, trying to identify children with health issues who aren't succeeding in the classroom. The theory is that if those health challenges can be identified and properly treated or managed, important barriers to learning can be mitigated or eliminated.

And the data are staggering. Here's what CHF's health screening teams found: Among the nearly two thousand children who comprise the total student body in the three schools, 23 percent had unrecognized or unmanaged vision problems requiring glasses, or if they had a pair, the prescription was out of date. Another 10 percent had hearing problems. While the percentage of children with visual challenges is about 20 percent nationally, more than 95 percent of nonpoor children are diagnosed early and get the correction they need.

Many children sat in classrooms with asthma out of control. According to a 2015 CHF survey, in South Bronx's P.S. 49, one in five children suffered with asthma; in P.S. 140, nearly a third of the children, 31 percent, were reported as having this most common of pediatric chronic illnesses. P.S. 140 is the school where the principal must call 911 at least weekly to bring a child with uncontrollable wheezing and coughing to a local emergency room. Just as a reference point, the overall national percentage of children diagnosed with asthma is less than 9 percent.

Kids languish in these poverty-filled classrooms. Teachers reported some 13 percent of their students were experiencing dental pain on any given day. Even more alarming were teacher reports that more than one in four (28 percent) of their students regularly experienced hunger.

And it's not just purely medical challenges, pain and hunger, that hold so many poor children back. The CHF surveys of the three pilot schools indicated that between 15 and 20 percent of the elementary school students showed signs of depression, anxiety, or stress. Many more—some 29 percent of a smaller sample of children—exhibited "disruptive behaviors." Many teachers and parents feel powerless to manage these issues as they erupt in the classroom, spilling over from lives in the shelters or the squalid apartments of neighborhoods in distress where adversity is prevalent and opportunity seems entirely elusive.

Most of us don't know these schools, don't walk in these neighborhoods, don't see the faces of these children, don't feel the anxieties and fears of their parents, can't taste the hopelessness that eventually replaces too many of the dreams that are the natural and appropriate aspirations of any child. But when the possibilities for these children are constricted, the inevitable outcome is another generation of unforgiving adversity and unfulfilled dreams—so bad for these smiling kids in P.S. 140's cafeteria and terrible, too, for America's future.

PART II
Roots

Brooklyn Baby, Coatesville Kid

Even anticipating the shocked feedback from the hipster nation of Brooklyn, New York, I need to be upfront about the community of my birth: I never really developed any particular affinity for the place. Why would I have? I lived there as a baby, and again as an eleven-year-old in the remote Brooklyn neighborhood of Fort Hamilton, home to a VA hospital where my father worked. Of interest to me was the fact that Fort Hamilton was—and still is—an active military installation where active-duty U.S. Army personnel were stationed. This meant that kids were allowed to play in the abandoned artillery bunkers and had access to the PX and to the movie theater on the base. For twenty-five cents we could see an afternoon's worth of main features, a slew of cartoons, "shorts," and a newsreel. That was all fine, but not enough to make me a die-hard Brooklyn Dodger fan or care one way or another whether we stayed in the borough or left when my father was "let go" from the VA because, as my mother once whispered to me, "he wouldn't fill out the forms they required and he was *always* making trouble."

My personal reservations notwithstanding, there's a lot to be said for Brooklyn, especially its history of adapting to wave upon wave of immigrants who saw the borough as the gateway to America, coming in droves to find jobs and raise their children in the clusters of prideful ethnic neighborhoods, always overlapping and ever shifting. Brooklyn, where the miracle of gentrification lifted once threatening, dangerous neighborhoods like Red Hook and Williamsburg into some level of grace and desirability, even though only the upwardly mobile can now afford the rents.

I spent the first year of my life with my maternal grandparents, Sylvia and Charlie, in their tiny third-floor walk-up apartment centrally located in Brooklyn's Flatbush neighborhood. The apartment barely accommodated the two of them, but my grandparents never thought twice about squeezing in my mother and me just because our options were limited. My father, Joe, who had already served with the U.S. Army in Europe, was, by 1944, stationed in California, waiting for the orders that would send him to Japan as part of the great Allied invasion and defeat of that country. When the invasion was deferred because of the atomic bombings of Hiroshima and Nagasaki in August 1945, Joe found a small cottage in Venice, California. My mother and I headed west, the family together for the first time, where my brother Neil was born in 1948, and then on to rural Pennsylvania, where Joe would be employed as a psychologist at the local VA hospital.

I had just turned five and Neil was a year old when we settled first on the top floor of a farmhouse in Wagontown, a hamlet in Chester County forty-five miles due west of Philadelphia. That lasted less than a year, almost through kindergarten, until we moved to another farmhouse, bigger and older than the first one, although we still couldn't afford to rent more than half of the place.

The one-room schoolhouse I attended accommodated the few local students in each of the six elementary grades, all taught by one teacher—decidedly not the usual educational venue for kids born in Brooklyn. Using an outdoor privy, getting water from a pump down the road, and fetching coal from the cellar in a tin bucket for the potbellied stove were all part of that strange reality.

So was the process for academic evaluation and advancement. Mrs. Neighbor taught in the school where I was attending second grade. Two months into the school year, she sent me home with a handwritten note to my mother that read something to the effect of "Irwin is an excellent reader. I want to move him to the third grade row. Do I have your permission?" My mother clearly remembered the incident and said she wrote one word, "yes," on the note and instructed me to return it to Mrs. Neighbor. Dutifully, I did. That same day, I was unceremoniously moved from the second graders' row to join the third graders. I would be surprised if any of my classmates even noticed that the "good reader" had changed seats. It hardly made a difference to me, either.

When the system finally consolidated, each of the one-room, six-grade/six-row schools now served a single grade. It was a revolutionary change in this isolated backwater, but as an eight-year-old, I'm sure that I didn't think twice about it. After all, young children have no frame of reference, other than their own living circumstances at any given moment. For a long time, it all seemed just normal: living in half a farmhouse on a country road in rural Pennsylvania, being able to wander down to the active dairy cow barn, once even exposed to the visual trauma of a veterinarian "treating" a cow for constipation. Without going into details, suffice it to say that he had to wear a rubber glove that went up to his shoulder. No one ever asked me, but if someone had, I would have assumed that watching the vet assist that moaning cow would be something all kids observed every now and then.

We didn't question it at the time, but I never understood precisely why we lived in that depressed rural farming community during my early elementary school years. My younger brother Neil and I just lived where we lived, went to the school we were taken to at the beginning of the year, and that was that.

Business as usual in the old farmhouse meant dealing with flying squirrels in the chimney, bats in the attic, an occasional escaped cow in the backyard, and whatever else was part of the day-to-day in a rented farmhouse. Our particular lives were all we knew; circumstances beyond our control. That same "it is what it is" reality goes for all children—those of the highly affluent and those who drift around in an urban shelter system. It is true for children who are emotionally or physically abused, and even for the children of addicts and crisis refugees. This is the life they know. Sometimes, for some kids there is adaptation and an inherent ability to survive and thrive, no matter what.

These children, the ones who persist and succeed, we call "resilient"; the ones who are trying to cope with deprivation, disparities, and fear we call "vulnerable" and "at risk." My family was never really honest-to-God poor, though we struggled. Financial grumblings were frequent and intense. For the most part, we lived in an environment of emotional instability and an odd kind of learned self-reliance which, as I look back, was a skill set that served my brothers and me well in the decades to come.

Eric Gary, my youngest brother, was born in the summer of 1952. The whole thing was shrouded in mystery, like so much else during that era when it was generally thought that everything possible should be done to keep children out of loop. Neil was just four and I was about to turn eight.

Mom was pregnant; that much we knew. When she went into labor, our father drove her the three-and-a-half miles from Wagontown to a hospital in Coatesville. Thelma, the other tenant sharing our house, was left in charge. We were told that Mom needed to go to the hospital so that the doctors could "get the baby out"—but not to worry, she would be home in a few days (turned out to be ten very long days)

Neil and I couldn't get past the notion of "getting the baby out," each of us having some sort of highly distorted picture in our heads about the reality of a baby "in there" in the first place. Neither of us would dare ask too many questions, but out of childhood curiosity I am certain that we would have appreciated knowing just what the doctor was actually going to do to help with the arrival of our baby brother. I didn't have any kind of usable mental image of a hospital that I could bring to mind to help make sense of any of this.

The following year, it all got real when a persistent ear infection with a high fever landed me at the same hospital for a weeklong stay. Nowadays, ear infections are diagnosed in the doctor's office, and from the 1960s through the 1990s, the condition was treated with a simple prescription. A big breakthrough came in 1985, when a new vaccine was introduced that protects children against the bacteria *Haemophilus influenzae* type b (Hib), not only a major cause of serious ear infections but also responsible for a lethal form of meningitis and other serious complications.

However, the situation for me as a nine-year-old patient in a ward filled with cribs and hospital beds was clearly memorable—and not in a good way. In a nutshell, I was feeling lousy, I was terrified, and I missed my mother. Visiting hours, much like in San Quentin, was limited to an hour a day and strictly enforced. Parents only. Sixty years later I can still see the overweight, profoundly unpleasant morning nurse scowling at me.

"Sit up!" she would snarl. "Look at this mess you've made with these rumpled sheets and your pillow on the floor."

Upset and embarrassed, trying hard not to cry, all I could think about was the visit from my mother that would happen at 3:00 p.m. sharp every day. The important point of all this whining about an event that occurred decades ago is simply that I never forgot how *unnecessarily* agonizing the experience was for me. On the clinical rotations in pediatrics as a medical student in Miami, as a resident in training, as the director of a pediatric intensive care unit, as the pediatrician in the dregs and despair of Lee County, Arkansas, as a visitor to the children's wards of hospitals in rural Honduras and famine-stricken Ethiopia, and as a doctor for thousands of New York's homeless children, I never forgot what it felt like as a nine-year-old boy hospitalized in Coatesville, Pennsylvania.

Every experience I had seems to have reinforced a fundamental truth about caring for vulnerable people, especially for children who live with terrible adversity for much of their childhood: empathy and compassion for vulnerable people is the starting point for a career—and a life—committed to caring for children.

In a way, I'm grateful to Nurse Ratchett, or whatever her name was, who in 1953 made sure that I was as miserable as possible in the children's ward of that hospital in Coatesville. I finally got to symbolically stick it to her almost fifty years later when we opened the Children's Hospital at Montefiore in October 2001. I was the lead designer and ultimately president of what was considered one of the most innovative and family-centered institutions in the country.

In my remarks at the opening of the hospital, just weeks after the World Trade Center terror attacks, I made the point that this beautiful new children's hospital was a symbol of hope and pride, essentially an antidote to the horrors of 9/11. Though I kept it to myself, sitting up there on the dais with hospital bigwigs, the mayor of New York City, and freshman senator Hillary Rodham Clinton, waiting my turn to speak, I remembered that agonizing week as a nine-year-old patient, knowing that nobody even remotely like that nurse in Coatesville would ever get through the door of my new children's hospital.

For many years, I never had a clear understanding about how or why Joe and Charlotte Redlener, two children in tow, one on the way, ended up in Wagontown, when by any definition we were hard-core city people. Long after my father died, all was revealed. The old man had infuriated boss after boss in one VA hospital after another. Finally, he got an ultimatum: "Your last shot is this facility in Pennsylvania. Don't screw it up!" As it turned out, he did screw it up, though it wasn't his last shot at all.

Over time, I had a vague but growing sense of being different. As nonobservant and detached from Judaism as we were, we were occasionally reminded that, for the good people of Chester County, Pennsylvania, Jews were quite the oddity. Never actually discriminated against or actively shunned, at least as far as my brothers and I were aware, we were socially isolated in a place where we were welcomed but never truly included in the social and cultural rhythm of the community.

One of my mother's most repeated stories, delivered with gusto for anybody who would listen, concerned my first day in fourth grade. The teacher was waiting outside the schoolhouse greeting the clean-shirted, neatly dressed nine-year-olds, shaking hands with the parents, smiling at the new students. Charlotte pulled our old Studebaker up onto the dirt driveway, waving as we got out of the car, and waited in line to meet the teacher.

"Oh, yes, I've been looking forward to meeting you," said the teacher looking at my mother, then me. I was already anxious when the teacher put her hand on my head, rubbing and feeling my scalp for what seemed like a strangely prolonged amount of time. In the awkwardness of that moment, I said nothing, of course, but my mother, clearly not comfortable with whatever was going on, and being a woman never, ever described as reticent or timid, said, "Excuse me, but what are you doing?"

Sweet, smiling, and seemingly innocent, the teacher said, "Oh, I just wanted to feel his little horns. I know that you're a Jewish family and that the boys have horns." My mother was aghast and explained that this was just a fable, a silly myth. Then, as I was still trying to process this strangest of conversations, Charlotte leaned down, gave me a peck on the cheek, and hurried off, back to the car. I was left rattled and anxious in a strange place where I would never forget that *I was different*, a feeling that never really left me and was, indeed, regularly reinforced throughout my child-hood and adolescence.

I had my good days in Chester County, too, minor triumphs that on some level endeared me to my classmates and the teachers. During the Korean War years in the early 1950s, Americans were encouraged to organize what were known as "scrap drives," the idea being to find discarded items made of tin or other metal. All of it would be collected by the government and moved to found-ries, where the metals could be recycled into weapons, ammuni-tion, and other needs of the war machine.

Our little rural schools competed to see which classroom could salvage the most usable metal, the winner being honored during a celebratory parade in Coatesville, the county seat. Schools that did well would be lucky to have collected a few hundred pounds of tin cans and small pieces of machinery.

I dramatically raised the stakes in this small town display of unity and patriotism by what could only be described as an extraordinarily serendipitous, if not downright miraculous, find. It seems that on the field just beside our rented farmhouse apart-ment, obscured from the road by a clump of trees, was a terri-bly rusted old bulldozer, clearly abandoned long ago, until I, an eight-year-old kid trying to play along, to fit into an environment that was as foreign to me and my family as being suddenly trans-ported to the Far East would have been, whose head was searched for horns by my own teacher, became the local hero by finding a nearly two-ton bulldozer and, with this grand discovery, blow-ing away any and all competition in our scrap drive contest. My mother didn't need much time to convince our farmer landlord that he, too, would be making a contribution to America's efforts to stop the Chinese aggression on the Korean Peninsula, if only Irwin was allowed to claim the machine in his fourth-grade effort to dominate that year's scrap drive.

"Of course he can," recalled my mother of her conversation with the farmer.

Done and done. Officials showed up with a flatbed truck and a winch—and off went the bulldozer to be weighed and celebrated as a great find.

I was the hero, the giant slayer who was responsible for the overwhelming victory that for the remainder of the school year became a point of pride for my classmates and our teacher. When the end-of-drive parade was finally organized in Coatesville, there we were, first in the lineup, with gap-toothed, hornless Irwin Elliot Redlener at the front of the pack, carrying the American flag, looking for all the world like that was precisely where he belonged.

For reasons now entirely obscure, my classmates elected me school chaplain, which I knew was meant to be an honor, perhaps a reward for dominating the scrap drive. I was terrified of what that might—and actually did—entail. To begin with, I had to read a portion of the New Testament every morning, a task that was a cause of great anxiety. Even though my knowledge of Jewish heritage and religious tenets was limited, I was, nonetheless, terrified that the God of Abraham was going to strike me dead for reading, *out loud*, the teachings of Jesus Christ. The upshot was that this was yet another childhood experience that ultimately forced me to face an unavoidable conclusion: I was *different*.

My father, a complex, emotional roller-coaster ride for his wife and children, capable of loving, funny moments, of occasional drunkenness, of fits of rage, of hard-left political positions and mysterious relatives who lived in the Catskill Mountains, where they would gather with other like-minded, marginalized Jews who regularly reminisced about the good old days in mother Russia, all the while waiting for the coming revolution that would bring America to its senses, ushering in another socialist state where the common good, as defined by a people's government, prevailed by decree and unanimous consent.

Joe was as capable of great kindness as he was prone to outbursts, the latter mostly directed at our mother, herself no pushover, scaring us half to death when she refused to back down, pushing and pushing the old man's rage buttons. I assume we learned something about courage and strong women, even as we feared, with good reason, a physically violent outcome to the big battle over how much was spent on our new clothes for the coming school year.

The two of them lacked any compunction in physically going after my brothers and me for real or perceived infractions that ranged from calling each other names to physical fighting or more ambiguous deviations that we might not have fully understood. Admittedly, I didn't think much of it at the time, but we were physically punished on a regular basis by both parents, occasionally with a few whacks from a leather belt just for emphasis.

Joe had been an infantry soldier during World War II. Only after his death in 1976 did we find a small cache of photos he had taken during the liberation of a German concentration camp. They were the kind of images, small black-and-white photos, I had dwelled on with horror during my teenage years when I became an avid reader, obsessed with the insanities of the Holocaust. I mourned the death of my father, but was beyond frustrated that I never had the opportunity to know about, no less discuss with him, precisely how those wartime experiences had affected him.

I eventually learned that his military career was a wild ride of advance and retreat, though not on the battlefield. A brilliant, college-educated man who had no tolerance for authority, clearly ill-suited for the hierarchy of the U.S. Army, the old man lived in an unending cycle of promotions from buck private to corporal, back to private, up to staff sergeant, back down to private. His superiors were alternately impressed with his brilliance, snatching him from an artillery unit to be trained as a German-speaking translator and interrogator, then, disgusted by his refusal to respect the order of things or the authority of his superiors, demoting him again and again for insubordination.

Who knows what he saw or what he did when he and his fellow soldiers fought their way into those hell camps? The images in

Dad's photos showed the gaunt faces of terribly emaciated survivors and piles of human corpses. It would be hard to understand what impact that experience would have on this good-looking, volatile psychologist who eventually went to work for the Veterans Administration after the war. This was decades before posttraumatic stress disorder was described. Expressions like "shell-shocked" were in vogue—not that I think that would be anywhere close to describing the impact of what the troops saw in the working death camps like Auschwitz, Buchenwald, Dachau, and so many others.

Joe was a secular Jew with a never fully explained disdain for rabbis. He mocked anything he deemed "mainstream" and distrusted government. He became a veteran with a grudge who engaged himself deeply in anti–Vietnam War protests and the struggles for civil and human rights until the day he died in 1976. He went to the marches and the rallies and supported the most progressive candidates. He was targeted by the infamous Senator Joe McCarthy and his House Un-American Activities Committee, eventually losing his job as a psychologist in the VA system, only to be reinstated nine months later when his indefatigable wife wrote to dozens of federal government officials demanding that Joe get his job back.

In the fog of childhood, my brothers and I, pretty much unaware of the context of Dad's turn of fortune, did think it curious that for that brief period he was a door-to-door salesman peddling Fuller brushes (all sizes, shapes, and functions) in the neighborhood. We looked in his sample case and were certainly curious, but for the most part we were impressed that our father had a new a job that was a lot easier to understand than whatever it was he did at the VA hospital. Still, his violent outbursts, mostly directed at our mother, occasionally at us, seemed to be increasingly frequent, always unpredictable, triggered by the most unimportant acts of commission or omission, unleashing demons that kept us in a constant state of anxiety, never knowing when the lid would blow off.

Good times? Yes, there were those, just hardly ever when the five of us were together. Our parents would be in the front seat of the family car, looking straight ahead, screaming at each other about keeping the window open or closed, or missing a turn, or when, in a rage, my father threw a bottle of ketchup, smashing it on the wall above my head in our small kitchen, or my mother accusing him of putting me in grave danger by insisting that I help him carry a washing machine down to the basement.

No dispute was too small for battle, no conflict forgotten, for Charlotte and Joe, the Brooklyn beauty and the handsome soldier she had married on an Army base in Boca Raton, Florida, on a lovely day in March 1943—a moment captured in a black-and-white photo of the smiling couple on the steps of the military chapel.

In 1955 he was transferred again, this time to the Fort Hamilton Veterans Administration Hospital in Brooklyn, New York, truly now his very last opportunity to make it in a system that he loathed and where the feeling was apparently mutual. Why he stayed and kept trying to make a go of it, we never knew. We could only imagine that it was his insecurity about making a living and that the predictability of the government system was probably some comfort even for a guy who never felt part of that system— or any other. It was tough, but, for the time being, we were back in Brooklyn, my birthplace, though a community where I felt as out of place as I did in the midst the farms and Christian culture of Coatesville, Pennsylvania.

Then, academic lightning struck. I was a perfectly happy fifth grader in Public School 106 when my teacher, the beloved Carl Geraci, told the principal that young Irwin didn't really need to pass through sixth grade and should be immediately skipped to seventh. I wish I could say that this fateful decision was driven by somebody's sense that they were dealing with a budding genius. Alas, as far as we knew, there was no such evidence, at least none shared with me or my parents. My hunch is that whatever I did

to adapt to a tumultuous, bizarre, and occasionally violent childhood must have endowed me with some kind of life skills that
looked like higher intelligence. I'll never know.

What I do know is that with this additional grade skipping
(I had already skipped second grade back in Wagontown), I was
now the youngest kid in my class, socially out of it throughout
the rest of my school years, and decidedly not ready for college
when I graduated from high school at fifteen. I was nice enough, I
suppose—but not ready for the big time, academically or socially.
The fact is that I was pretty much an average student, and neither
my parents nor I ever really understood why I was skipped at all.

The path from that point to medical school was complicated;
at once exhilarating and surreal, the journey was definitely convo-
luted and, in a way, fascinating. The process took me from Long
Island to Ohio to Belgium to Miami, where the vaunted "MD"
was finally granted. By that that time, at the end of a winding
academic road, I was in the game and focused.

My father was sixty when he suffered a massive hemorrhagic
stroke while sleeping in his home in upstate New York, going
into a deep coma from which he never recovered. I was a thirty-
two-year-old physician already on the faculty of the University of
Miami Medical School. I am pretty sure I was an accomplice, an
inadvertent material contributor, to my father's demise, an enabler
who listened to his ranting complaints about the care he was getting for his uncontrollable hypertension, his latent diabetes, and
his ulcers.

"Jesus Christ, Irwin!" He'd yell into the receiver. "That son of
a bitch gave me this new medication, and I know it won't work.
Could kill me. Send me the PDR sheet on this," referring to the
Physician's Desk Reference, a comprehensive information source
on all available medications, written for practicing physicians.
"I'm not taking these goddamn pills until we really check it out."

Dutifully, I did what he asked. I'd send him the source material,
and he would peruse the details, look for the rare complications

and side effects—and not take the medications. Sometimes he was right. Sometimes I had to agree that his doctor had actually prescribed a drug that was just wrong.

More often than not, he would go back to his doctor and berate him for not paying attention to what was being prescribed. Meanwhile, his blood pressure and blood sugar were out of control, conditions that led inexorably to the bursting of a small artery on the left side of his brain. Maybe I should have stood my ground and told my father to listen to his doctor's advice. Then again, years later, it was reported that one of the new drugs prescribed for my father's diabetes was responsible for a high incidence of hemorrhagic strokes in adults with preexisting hypertension. Maybe Dad was right.

There is no question that growing up with Joe and Charlotte Redlener was regularly, though not always, traumatic and unsettling for my brothers and me. Yet the three of us turned out to be reasonably sane, neatly situated somewhere along that wide spectrum of normal, successful adults. How does that happen? How do some children emerge successfully from childhood traumas, and others do not?

There are two key factors at work. First is that some children are born with high levels of resiliency—genetically influenced coping skills and the ability to self-regulate emotional responses to stressful situations. A second factor is being fortunate enough to have at least one core relationship that helps buffer a child from the most severe consequences of stress and trauma. This protector can be a parent or another caretaker, sometimes a grandparent or even an older sibling. In the case of the Redlener boys, it was all about Momma Charlotte, a pillar of strength, consistency, love, and support that never wavered. That's an emphatic *never* that lasted until she lay on her deathbed in the hospital, reaching out to her grown sons whom she protected and nurtured through every storm of our turbulent childhoods and the trials, big and small, of adult life, too.

A Winding Road from College to Med School

Having graduated from high school three months before my sixteenth birthday, I wasn't exactly ready for college, though I was accepted at Drew University, a small school in Madison, New Jersey. Freshman year was a mini-disaster, academically and socially, including incidents involving pellet guns, driving a girlfriend's MG convertible on and off campus without a license, refusing to attend chapel, and a general reputation of not exactly taking the college experience all that seriously, at least not in the considered opinion of the Methodist seminarians whose presence throughout the long history of Drew University dominated the campus. Suffice it to say, I was invited not to return for sophomore year.

Now what? The matriarch insisted that I apply to other schools immediately and "strongly suggested" that I not reveal that I had been dropped by Drew, instead claiming that I had been "traveling" that year after high school graduation. I was offended by my own mother's encouraging me to lie on a college application!

"No! That's not right," I said, defiantly including the wayward Drew experience on the application to Adelphi University. I was promptly rejected. That was enough of a wake-up call. When I applied to Hofstra University in Hempstead, New York, there was no mention of Drew. The letter of acceptance arrived a couple of weeks later.

Hofstra in 1961 was a commuter-only school, which was just fine for me. Dorms were nonexistent, and graduate programs were few and far between. Years later I watched with pride as the school grew under the dynamic leadership of its latest president, Stuart Rabinowitz. By 2015 there were dorms, a law school, a new medical school, and more.

My parents had divorced in 1960, and by the time I started classes at Hofstra, my mother was teaching sixth grade in the particularly affluent Long Island community of Great Neck, where the cost of living far exceeded anything we could afford. So we rented a walk-up "on the other side of the tracks" in Little Neck, Queens, one of New York City's outer boroughs. I made my way back and forth to Hofstra by car pool, bus, or when it was available, my mother's old Chevy.

I was more or less "pre-med" at Hofstra, with a major in psychology. The thought of going to medical school was on the list of possibilities, but I was deeply distracted, in spite of the fact that Charlotte had been pushing the idea of "my son, the doctor" while I was still in diapers.

In general, my experience at Hofstra was, putting it kindly, "eclectic." I was indeed pre-med, but worked for more than a year trying to organize a national magazine for university students. I also thought, albeit briefly, about becoming a dentist and considered changing my major from psychology/pre-med to history. Then there was brief flirtation with a possible career in the military and an actual attempt to enlist in the Navy to be trained as a fighter pilot. The entry process included a full day of testing at the old Floyd Bennett Field, an operating base for the New York Air National Guard located on a small island just off the coast of Brooklyn. I failed the spatial orientation tests.

"OK," said the reviewer, "you're never going to fly our airplanes, but would you be interested in getting a commission to be trained in naval air intelligence?"

No, thanks.

Then there was my brief, though intense, foray into publishing. In my junior year at Hofstra, I met another student who, as a twenty-year-old, had an assumed name, a kind of nom de plume, that he was "trying out," but ultimately retained. Somehow that felt strangely exotic. I have no idea what his real name was, but I knew him as Michael Bruce. Michael was working hard on starting a magazine that would directly target U.S. college and university students. At the time, nothing like that existed, and I was very intrigued, agreeing to partner with young Mr. Bruce in his quest to create a new magazine we called *Dawn*.

With a little personal money, Michael rented us a run-down, loft-like office on lower Fifth Avenue in Manhattan, somehow acquiring rudimentary furniture and printing business cards for both of us. We started from scratch but got much further than I could have guessed we would. The great writer Gay Talese, then a staff writer for *Esquire*, more or less took me under his wing, offering practical advice and lots of useful contacts. Among other favors, Talese connected us with *Esquire*'s art director, who did the cover photography for *Dawn*'s first issue. We got pretty far along in this adventure, including landing interviews with Ray Charles, Joan Baez, famed comedian and social commentator Dick Gregory, and others, but at the end of the day, long before crowdsourcing was an option, we couldn't raise the money to actually launch the magazine. And that was that.

As my career plans drifted from medicine to jet fighter pilot to magazine publishing, Charlotte was increasingly unhappy and determined to "keep hope alive" that her eldest son would one day return to his senses and become the doctor every Jewish mother dreamed about as her son's manifest destiny. In the winter of my senior year at Hofstra, she dragged me out to a hospital on Long Island, just east of the city. She was intent on introducing me to an emergency medicine physician there who had attended medical school at the Catholic University of Louvain in Belgium, an ancient, highly regarded European institution that taught classes in both French and Flemish. (Belgium is a divided country with two distinct cultures and political systems that, incidentally, never really got along very well. The southern part of Belgium is populated principally by the French-speaking Walloons; to the north are the Flemish-speaking Flamands. In the middle was the Catholic University of Louvain, which taught in both languages and was immersed, oddly enough, in both cultures.)

Phil, the slim, balding American who had graduated from Louvain, sang the school's praises and urged me to apply—at least as a backup, an option my mother demanded that I pursue. I agreed, got the paperwork, and sent it in—then promptly and entirely forgot that I had ever done so.

There were other adventures on the horizon following graduation from Hofstra. Because I had been rejected from the handful of American med schools I had applied to, everything was on the table.

In the late spring of 1964, with graduation looming and just before turning twenty, notions of becoming a magazine publisher, joining the Navy, or going to medical school were all pretty much out of mind. Nonetheless, I was revved up just thinking about possible next moves, a state of mind that my parents couldn't understand, and, in a rare moment of spousal agreement, they let me know that they disapproved of "drifters without direction," as my father (of all people) characterized what they both feared would happen to their oldest son.

Children in Jail

While there were indeed options on the table, I ended up joining a new program sponsored by the U.S. Department of Labor called Project Cause. The central idea was to train young people, mostly recent college graduates, to work with inner-city youth and staff economic development programs in struggling communities, a notion that aligned well with my own interests in doing something of value, perhaps even an ode to my father and his lefty outlaw uncles and their coconspirators in the mountains of upstate New York.

The experience with Project Cause, based at the time on the campus of Ohio University in Athens, Ohio, turned out to be far more important in shaping my attitudes and personal aspirations than I could have imagined. Toward the end of the first month of training, the new trainees were told that each of us would be sent out to spend a day observing at a local agency serving vulnerable children. I was up for the idea and highly intrigued when I was driven by Ralph, one of the program supervisors, to a facility described as a "residential unit for troubled children," or something to that effect. The translation of that turned out to be "reform school," where children and youth were incarcerated for a period of weeks to years.

"You mean, this is a *jail*?" I asked Ralph as we rode up to the main entrance.

"Well, you might say something like that, I guess," the supervisor responded. "Just don't pass any judgments until you see what goes on here. It's supposed to be not too bad. Really geared toward treating and supporting troubled kids."

"Sure," I said hopefully.

Once inside, we got a personal tour led by one of the institution's social workers. She seemed nice enough, but as we got deeper into the place, it was clear that this in no way felt like a support center. We walked through the drab yellow corridors, past office after office, on to the locked areas where the congregate sleeping wards were located, each of which appeared to contain some twenty to thirty cots. No children were in the ward we walked through. I did see neatly folded clothes on many of the cots, some obviously belonging to very young kids. There were bars on the windows, and as I looked out to a grassy quad, I saw a couple of dozen children being watched by a handful of adults. A few of the children were playing kick ball; others, mostly older—looking twelve to fifteen years of age or so—were milling around.

"It's free exercise time," the social worker offered, though we hadn't asked.

Ralph and I were allowed to peek into the bathroom, which served the needs of at least two sleeping wards. The place was clean but deeply impersonal; rows of toilets without so much as separation or privacy barriers, unraveling rolls of toilet paper randomly on the floor between the commodes.

We walked silently out into the hallway, the place feeling increasingly cold and intimidating. Passing an open office door, I heard what sounded like a child whimpering and looked into what seemed to be an anteroom, where I saw a child sitting on a small sofa next to an older man—probably in his fifties—who was speaking softly to the boy. Neither noticed me in the doorway.

"Please come back out here," our social worker tour guide said to me, considerably more stern than she had been as we were walking through the facility.

"OK," I said, "but what's going on?"

"That," the social worker said, "is a young man who is *always* in trouble—never listens and always breaking the rules. I guess that's why he's here."

"How old is he?"

"Six. He'll be seven next month, I believe."

"Do these kids get some kind of treatment while they're here?"

"Treatment? We do what we can, but they're here mostly for disciplinary reasons."

The reality of this situation hit like a gut punch. The idea of a six-year-old boy in what I saw as a prison was roiling me. I didn't totally appreciate it at the time, but I was memory banking an experience that would stay with me. *A first grader in jail?* This was deeply disconcerting on so many levels, though at that very moment I couldn't really process what it all meant, no less what should be done about it. I just knew that there was something terribly wrong here in southeast Ohio, in this isolated facility where a small child was getting a dressing-down from a man who, I imagined, had no idea how crazy it was for a little boy to be in what, for all intents and purposes, seemed to be nothing more than a jail for little children.

I asked Ralph if we could go back to the campus in Athens. I'd had enough. I think he felt the same way.

It was just a month later, well into my summer training for Project Cause, that I received a phone call from my mother.

What? Did You Say *Belgium?*

"Great news, my boy," she exuded, "you've been accepted to medical school."

"What? Where?" I said, thinking that one of the U.S. schools that initially rejected me had finally come to its senses and reconsidered my application.

"In Louvain. You know, that medical school in Belgium."

I was silent, soaking in this news and trying to figure out exactly what to say, but before I had a chance to organize my response, Mom said, "I sent you a bus ticket. See you tomorrow night."

Two weeks later I was on an Icelandic Airlines turboprop flying from New York to Luxembourg—the cheapest flight available. I was nineteen and had never been out of the country, and now I had to find my way through Europe, identify a place to live, and enroll in a medical school where English was not an option. In spite of it all, I could not have been more excited.

With minimal instructions in hand, I found the correct train from the airport in Luxembourg to Louvain, Belgium. I had an address of a small hotel, the Majestic, where I was to stay until I could identify student housing. I was exhausted but fully charged up when I disembarked at the main train station in Louvain. Well before the era of roller luggage, all of my possessions were packed into two large suitcases. Fortunately, the Majestic was a straight half-mile trek down Avenue des Allies. The walk set the stage perfectly. It was the real deal: block after block of historic stone buildings with carved facades and classic European shops open for business and bustling.

Arriving at the Majestic, my instructions were to ask for Madame Marie, the proprietress. I walked into the lobby, which led directly to the café's dining room. Off to the right was a massive wooden reception desk, mailboxes, and hooks holding the room keys on the wall behind. The place was classic old European, and I was absorbing it all when the Madame approached, hand extended, smiling and welcoming. Dressed simply in a floral skirt and blouse, I guessed her to be in her early fifties.

"Bonjour, monsieur!"

I responded as best I could in my lame excuse for French, but I did learn that the reservation my mother had made was actually booked and ready. Before even getting to the paperwork, I absorbed everything I could about the look of the room. Round tables, mostly unoccupied, were decked out with very French decorative floral patterned tablecloths; a few glass chandeliers hanging from the ceiling. To the left was a winding stairway leading to the rooms above. There was a bar in the back of the restaurant area where a few guys were standing around drinking glasses of beer and laughing at some indecipherable inside jokes. A couple of young men I assumed were students glanced in my direction but kept their conversation going in the guttural sounds of Flemish, a dialect I never quite got used to.

My room was two floors up from the main floor and, once registered, Madame Marie handed me the large metal key and I went upstairs to unpack. An hour later I came back down for an early dinner of steak and fries, slathered with mayonnaise, a staple of Louvain and most of Belgium.

Getting into medical school in Belgium was nothing like the grueling, high-stress, competitive process applicants went through in the United States, where at least, once admitted, you were almost certain to graduate. Here, many students, Belgian and other nationals, including a large contingent of highly motivated Americans, were admitted more or less en masse. As at many academic counterparts across the continent, at Belgium's Catholic

University of Louvain, one of the oldest universities and medical schools in Europe, gaining admission was relatively perfunctory; staying in was another matter altogether. Less than 50 percent of the admitted class actually graduated from the six-year combined undergraduate and medical school program. Stress getting in versus stress staying in—pick your poison.

In the European model, which was certainly the case for Louvain, professors were distant and, particularly for the American students, seemingly unapproachable. The classes were taught in French or Flemish. In spite of my extremely undistinguished experience with French in high school and college, the Flemish option, rough and difficult, would have been unthinkable. So there I was, almost always sitting in the back row of a huge amphitheater, where I watched and listened to Professor Van Camp lecturing in French. Remarkably, as he lectured, using a different colored chalk in each hand, he sketched out the embryology of the central nervous system or whatever was the topic of the day.

Getting back to my small student room after classes, I would be exhausted but, after a short break, needed to hit the books. Sprawled out on my desk were my class notes, such as they were, the professor's formal course book, an English medical book on the topic, a French-English standard dictionary, and a French-English medical dictionary.

In accordance with long tradition, there were no exams during the academic year—in other words, no way to really know how one was doing. Formal classes were over by early May, with exams scheduled a month later. The gap, called "the block," was an intense four-week period during which students focused on getting ready for the exams. Some of us read and reread (and reread again) our notes and the various texts; others obsessively outlined the material. In other words, we tried to do whatever it took to memorize everything we had heard and seen in the teaching theaters and read in our study rooms throughout the preceding academic year, all the while realizing that some of us would fail and have to repeat the year or head back to wherever we came from.

After the block, we faced the feared and loathsome two weeks of one-on-one *oral* exams given individually by some pretty grumpy professors. After months of presentations, lectures, labs, and reading, only three questions might be asked. It was live or die right there and then, praying that the random questions presented to you were ones that you had actually studied and committed to memory.

"Décrivez l'os maxillaire, s'il vous plait (Describe the maxillary bone, please)," said the anatomy professor. OK, I thought, "I have this," and proceeded to describe every nook and cranny, every place where a major nerve or small artery passed through the large facial bone. There may have been twenty other bones that I couldn't have described if my life depended on it, but I lucked out that afternoon.

"Donnez-moi tous les dessins pour le développement du cœur (Give me all the drawings for the development of the heart)," sneered the cigar-puffing embryology Professor Van Camp. I sat across the small exam table, no more than thirty inches from the old man, who seemed to be purposefully gazing slightly upward, avoiding eye contact. Fine by me. Colored pencils and blank paper were in reach. The cigar smell was distracting, as was my own profuse sweating, but I pretty much knew what he was asking for and began to draw the series of seven stages of embryonic heart development.

I turned the paper around to show Van Camp my handiwork, when he slammed his fist onto the table, "Non!"

It seems I was unaware of the fact that Van Camp prided himself on being able to read upside down and didn't appreciate the innocent gesture of a young, highly intimidated American student.

The final reckoning came on a day in mid-June, with all two hundred or so of my classmates convening in one of the large meeting auditoriums. In a room offstage, all of our professors had gathered to sequentially and collaboratively review the test evaluations for each of us—one at a time. Meanwhile we all waited in the auditorium until the secretary of the faculty stepped out onto the stage and asked us to rise. Faculty filed in, taking their seats on the stage facing us. Then the secretary came forward to read each student's name in alphabetical order, follow by "Ajourner" (meaning defer or, in effect, fail) or "Passer" (you passed). Occasionally, the secretary would utter the golden words "Passer avec distinction," or great job. Once I heard the word "passer" after my name, everything else was a blur.

In the summer of 1965, between the first and second years in Louvain, I came home to New York, determined to marry my college girlfriend, Arlene Berman. We had spent the year I was away writing each other incessantly, usually three or four times a week, even getting engaged by mail. A week after the wedding, it was back to Louvain with my new bride in tow—and back to classes in an environment that remained foreign and intimidating for the three years I studied at Louvain. Yet somehow I survived the system and was ultimately able to organize a transfer to the third-year class at the University of Miami School of Medicine— the only U.S. medical school that would even consider a transfer application from a student in Belgium.

It was there in Miami that David Isaac was born in 1967. A wonderful life event, of course, but marred by the fact that fathers were just not permitted in the labor or delivery suites— in spite of the fact that I was a medical student at the time as well as "the father to be." We were shocked and dismayed, especially Arlene, who assumed I would be there to support her. I pulled every string I could to try circumventing that highly anachronistic rule, but to no avail. (Fortunately, by the time our second child, Jason Craig, was born in 1970 in New York, fathers were universally welcome and encouraged to participate in the process.)

After med school, I managed to secure a pediatric internship at Babies Hospital of Columbia-Presbyterian Hospital in northern

Manhattan. Now it was grown-up time. For that year, from July 1, 1969, to June 30, 1970, nothing else mattered beyond learning how to care for very sick children and coming of age as a doctor with a growing understanding of the importance of the so-called social determinants of health. That and an acute awareness of the social and political dynamics that were engulfing a turbulent American society in the early 1970s.

PART III
Real-World Medicine and Public Health

Lives in the Balance: The Real World of Internship

The graduation ceremony from medical school, the conferring of the MD degree in May 1969, was a landmark event to be sure, but not the big deal I had imagined. I don't know why that was the case. Part of the dynamic was a little anxiety about the reality of moving on to the internship; but maybe it all felt a little anticlimactic. In spite of my mother's over-the-top excitement, not to mention her feeling vindicated about pushing me so hard to become "my son, the doctor," there is something about formal ceremonies, especially my own, that I never much connected to. Glaring exceptions, of course, are the achievements, big and small, of my children and grandchildren.

The actual magic moment of transition for me, as for other newly minted doctors, happened on the first day of internship—when we step into that clinic or go to "work rounds" on the hospital wards and get our first patient assignments. Even though young doctors today work far fewer hours and are much more supervised than was the case when my cohort joined the profession, the fundamental thrill of that transition from student to doctor still holds. The reality of being responsible for the lives of other human beings who are medically fragile is a profound moment for physicians. I was no exception.

My first day of service as a pediatric intern included sign-off by the counterpart colleague I replaced. For each individual patient there would be an index card with basic information regarding vital statistics, diagnoses, lab results, and so on, and the course of events in the hospital, along with current clinical status, would be reviewed verbally in detail. Then *the* moment: standing with my team at the bedside of my first new patient and hearing something on the order of "Hi, Mrs. Jones. Please meet Dr. Redlener. He'll be taking over as your son's doctor."

Becoming an intern was in itself a unique and transformative human experience. But one of the realities that made that particular year so extraordinarily complex had to do with conditions *outside* the hospital, the impoverished Fort Washington community of new immigrants and underserved minorities who were united in their great ambivalence about the big ivory-tower teaching hospital where I now worked.

On the one hand, patients and families were mostly thankful for the care we delivered. On the other hand, many local residents deeply resented Columbia-Presbyterian Hospital for what they perceived as institutional arrogance and a deep disconnect between the hospital and the surrounding community. For every grateful patient, there seemed to be two who believed that the hospital exploited their relatives and neighbors, treating them as unwitting and vulnerable medical guinea pigs for young doctors to practice starting IVs and doing medical procedures or for professors to try out new medications and conduct clinical experiments. This backdrop of tension between the hospital and the community cast a shadow on everything we did and undermined shallow statements of concern regularly expressed by hospital officials.

Still larger social and political turmoil loomed outside the hospital wards and local community challenges. Even for overworked interns, there was no escaping the big-picture realities that demanded our attention, no matter what we were doing in the hospital. The evolving war in Vietnam, the sit-ins, the protests, and the continuing civil rights struggles engulfed the whole country. Conflict over Vietnam was ripping the nation apart, many of us not just questioning how the war would end but also worried about the political stability of the United States. Martin Luther King, Jr., and Bobby Kennedy had been assassinated the year before I started my internship.

On May 4, 1970, when National Guard troops killed four unarmed antiwar student protesters on the campus of Ohio's Kent State University, I harbored serious doubts about the United States' ability to survive these traumas intact. We seemed to have reached a breaking point where political and social positions were all but irreconcilable and national leadership had no exit strategy, not only for Southeast Asia but for the roiling discord at home. For me and many of my colleagues at Columbia-Presbyterian, the deadly Vietnam protests in Ohio breached a point of no return. As busy as we were working the wards and the ER, we couldn't stay out of the fray. So we took action.

In the immediate aftermath of the shooting, we organized a staff protest that culminated in a major rally on May 8 in the hospital's main auditorium. Keynote speaker Dr. Benjamin Spock, one of the nation's most vociferous and effective antiwar activists *and* a highly respected pediatrician and best-selling author of parent advice books on child rearing, was ill and unable to make it down from Boston. The night before the rally, he called me and dictated his intended remarks, asking me to deliver them on his behalf! It was a big deal, and I was honored to share his statement, which included these words: "*All of us must become activists to end the war . . . working in the current electoral campaigns, participating in demonstrations and confrontations. We in the health profession have a special responsibility.*"

Those words meant a lot. Here was a famed pediatrician, literally a household name known to every parent in America, but also a doctor who could not have been more public regarding his social and political beliefs. He was the first physician in modern times who sustained and enhanced his medical reputation while regularly speaking out and publicly demonstrating on the front lines of issues that went far beyond his professional expertise.

I wanted to be Spock.

One more extraordinary experience added to the emotional chaos of the year. On May 15, one week to the day after the hospital's Vietnam protest, my second son, Jason, was born. Arlene's obstetrician, Dr. Ed Bowe, was sure everything was fine. I waited in L & D (labor and delivery) with her and, when all was ready, accompanied the OB (obstetrics) team into the delivery suite, not expecting anything out of the ordinary. I was presumably there just for moral support—but as soon as Jason emerged, things took a terrifying turn. He was covered with meconium—stained amniotic fluid, a problem seen in babies who have been stressed during labor and delivery under circumstances such as constriction of the umbilical cord. He wasn't breathing, because he had aspirated some of the meconium, which now totally blocked his airway. My son was turning blue and did not respond to Dr. Bowe's rubbing his back or slapping his bottom.

I was watching this unfold with growing concern, maybe a bit of panic. I waited what seem like a very long time (but wasn't actually) for Bowe to do something effective. Finally, he did. The venerable OB doctor handed the struggling baby, my new son, to *me*!

"Here, do something!" he said.

No more thinking, no more delays. I put the baby on the treatment table in the delivery room, used suction to clear his airways, and began CPR. Thank God, it worked. I looked at Jason, his beautiful dark eyes lit up, finally breathing on his own and crying. I looked at Arlene, and she was in tears, too. I had saved my son's life and, in those few minutes, fell in love with him in a way that is impossible to describe, but unforgettable.

This, then, was the year of my internship: daily rounds, dying children and distraught parents, exhaustion from unending night call, deep dismay about America's stability, and trying to manage a marriage, a young son, and a baby on the way. That was a lot to process, and I was taking it all in, but compartmentalizing when I was dealing with patients, doing everything I could to stay focused on the clinical challenges at hand. Handling the unrelenting, self-generated internal pressures to provide the best possible medical care was about passion, the pursuit of excellence—and doing everything possible to function in the face of chronic fatigue. We all more or less persevered.

At the same time, coping with my growing concern about the world at large was, in its own way, deeply compelling and unsettling, certainly not easy to process. I wanted to protest our presence in Vietnam, and I was terrified about the killings of national leaders and students on an American college campus. But I still had to check out a new admission, wheezing badly and on her way up to the floor from the ER. After all, we were here to learn how to be doctors, no matter what was going on in Southeast Asia or in the community just outside the hospital doors.

For some in my demographic cohort—many in school or just entering the workforce or some still wandering, "searching for meaning," in the late 1960s and 1970s—there were overwhelming feelings of powerlessness in the face of widespread injustice or wrongheaded policies that led to inexplicable wars and domestic turmoil. In response, many young people became social activists and protesters; others "dropped out and turned on," sliding into a countercultural lifestyle of heavy drug use and disconnect.

Even issues like world hunger were absorbed into the never-ending, random streams of social consciousness that characterized certain kinds of activism in the 1970s. There were groups exhorting us to simply *declare* an end to world hunger—and that declaration alone would be all that would be needed to ameliorate the absence of stable access to nutritious food for the more than 200 million children experiencing malnutrition in developing countries in 1970.[1] This was another indulgent fantasy of First World dreamers, seemingly unable or unwilling to comprehend the hard challenges of really ending global hunger or poverty and inequity.

The same could be said of the people who feasted on the faddish "enlightenment" programs that peaked in California. They gathered by the thousands in movements like "est," a kind of populist cult that attracted followers apparently comfortable with an odd mix of passive acceptance of whatever they were told and tolerance for emotional and physical pain. Ultimately, est (Latin for "it is") was attacked by another group, Scientologists, who accused est founder Werner Erhard of stealing Scientology's ideas, originally expounded by that group's founder, L. Ron Hubbard, who believed that aliens from outer space had colonized the earth.

Then there were the Reichians, adherents of the philosophy taught by Wilhelm Reich, a twentieth-century "therapist" who focused on deep massages and improving sexual orgasms by collecting atmospheric "ions" in homemade blankets of steel wool.

All of this troubled me deeply. While American hedonists and hippies indulged themselves making orgasm-enhancing orgone blankets, children were indeed starving around the world, racism flourished in America, the scandals of Richard Nixon were emerging, and war was raging in Vietnam.

The Kent State incident was my own personal turning point. I eagerly volunteered to be one of the organizers of and speakers at a protest on the campus of my hospital. Energized and happy to address the packed audience, I spoke out against U.S. policies that seemed to be taking us to a terrible place of uncertainty and disruption, seemingly gutting our fundamental national values.

All of this activism had to coexist with my primary focus on caring for sick children in upper Manhattan, where the global travails of a planet groaning with troubles were hardly relevant. Life in the hippie communes, the bizarre cults of California, and young men dying in the Mekong Delta meant nothing whatsoever to the lives of most families struggling to survive amid the grinding poverty of a New York City ghetto.

The fact is that my job as a pediatric intern at New York's Columbia-Presbyterian Hospital demanded my full attention and insane hours—three or four all-night calls in the hospital every week, in addition to regular daytime duties. That reality limited my capacity to completely obsess about the constant stream of bad news from the outside world, though it was, to some degree, always on my mind.

Otherwise, internship was thrilling, disorienting, and often terrifying. Med school more or less taught the didactics of medical care, but, certainly at the beginning of the year, none of us seemed prepared to deal with this degree of responsibility for the life, death, and suffering of children and their families.

One entire ward of Babies Hospital was occupied by children with cancer. Many were just as sick from the cancer therapies of the time as they were from the malignancies that were killing them. We listened to the crying babies, saw the helpless sorrow of parents, the compassion of nurses, and, sometimes, the cold calculus of senior doctor-scientists who pushed every medicine, no matter the side effects or the near certain knowledge that recovery was simply out of the question. On an on went the meds, the lab tests, the writing of orders, the beeping monitors, the oblivion to the relentless suffering, until the patient expired, still attached to monitor leads and strapped to IV boards, barely able to receive a mother's hug.

It was not until decades later that "patient-centered care" concepts would demand that the feelings and needs of patients and their loved ones be major considerations in every aspect of medical care, including critical decisions about therapies, pain management, and comfort care. In the 1960s and 1970s, doctors were in tight control—sometimes bombastic, occasionally paternalistic, and ever righteous—making the decisions that would affect the health and well-being of every patient under their care.

For me and my intern cohort, this intense month of managing the care of children with terminal cancer may have been among the most difficult medical experiences of our careers. We would see these patients during the day, of course, and during the night if there was an acute need, but we also made three sets of "rounds" every day, all before noon. First, at a god-awful early morning hour, we saw patients, did a quick exam, talked to them and/or their parents, discussed problems, drew blood for testing, and checked on any results that might have come in during the night.

This first whirlwind around the ward was particularly hard for me. I was seeing these babies and children, strapped to IVs, many crying, some just out of it. This was unbearable for me for many reasons. I had my own young son at home, and on the rare occasions when I was actually there when he woke, the experience was pure joy.

But here in first rounds on the cancer ward, you walked into a sterile room and saw a child strapped down and wired up, usually whimpering, maybe still crying from the early blood drawing. Mom or Dad was standing at the bedside or sleeping in the chair in the corner of the hospital room, their eyes red, too. Sleep was fitful and filled with fears and anguish. They might be looking at me, but it was hard to tell exactly what was on their minds. I was committed to caring for their baby—and I wanted to care for them, too—but I was a twenty-five-year-old dad, a novice still learning the ropes of being a doctor, still unsure of exactly what to say that might provide a bit of comfort to a family who had no idea if their baby would live or die, worried about how much more suffering lay ahead in the days and weeks to come.

Second rounds were with our floor-supervising residents. We had to make sure the charts were up to date, with all clinical issues as resolved as they could be, all the while trying to soak up the wisdom of pediatric residents just a year or two ahead of us in the process. Blind leading the blind? Not really. It's difficult to overstate how much a young doctor in training learns in the course of a year. For the interns, the second- and third-year residents were generally effective mentors, certainly more experienced and knowledgeable than we were, and, for the most part, willing and able to share what they knew with us.

Our third set of rounds during our month on the children's cancer ward was with the *true* god: Professor James Wolff, MD, attending physician and well-known childhood cancer expert. It was on these "attending rounds" that we, the lowly house staff, presented our cases and were interrogated by *the* Dr. Wolff. Why did you get that test? What were the results of yesterday's tests? Why did the patient have that reaction? What are your plans for this patient now? Wolff was Socrates on the children's cancer ward.

Generally speaking, Wolff was brilliant and caring, a preeminent researcher responsible for many breakthroughs in the treatment of childhood leukemia, literally saving the lives of countless children with what had been considered an almost universally fatal disease.

Yet he was an enigma.

Compassionate as he was, rounding with him was difficult for many of us. He was a great teacher, and kindly to patients and their families, but he never relented in pushing the treatments for every child, every time. Many times we would see children whose conditions were truly terrible, suffering in pain, confined by restraints, vomiting, and visibly uncomfortable. It was obvious that a number of the children we saw on cancer rounds were just not going to make it, but Dr. Wolff pushed on anyway.

One day after rounds, I asked the professor if we could speak privately about his relentless treatment of all children, even those we all knew were not going to make it. Wouldn't it be more humane, even more reasonable medically, to make such decisions on an individual basis?

"Yes, we theoretically should take each case individually," Wolff responded. "But if I had to anguish over every child, every family, every day, I wouldn't last six months in this work. I decided years ago that I would just do everything available for every patient. I've already made the decision, preemptively. I'm not necessarily proud to say this, but it's the only way I could protect myself from being in a constant state of uncertainty—and needing to absorb the agony of every family. This is not a great answer, but it is the truth."

It was a short but sobering conversation about life and death decision making for critically ill children, even when "everyone" knew that the reality of the treatment was sometimes hardly better than the disease itself and the outcome, with or without the intense treatment, was generally uncertain. Still, the statistics were clear. Many more children with cancer were surviving as a direct result of Jim Wolff's discoveries.

For the medical students and residents in training, there was always an emotional toll in caring for children with terminal conditions. Jim Wolff was sufficiently self-aware to know that he had to protect himself, and he chose to do that by avoiding the daily decisions as much as he could. More chemo? Another IV? Of course, thought the great professor, we'll do whatever it takes to sustain the heartbeat and respirations.

The lessons we learned in those intimate engagements on the wards and in the clinics and emergency rooms were formative and indelible for everything that followed. Our patients came from the hard-core poverty neighborhoods in the far northern Manhattan communities of Washington Heights and Harlem, and we were schooled about what that meant for children and families awash in adversities.

The clinical experiences came quickly and furiously during what might be considered the late Wild West era of medical training. Since the 1980s, the working hours and conditions for medical students and doctors in training have been tightly regulated, as has legal and ethical responsibility for patient-care decisions; clinical orders written by trainees and students now must have a sign-off from the attending physician. For the most part, that's been a positive change, but "old school" internships, the kind of experience I went through, were a rite of passage through much of the twentieth century in American medical training programs.

Supervision for us medical greenhorns was minimal—and mostly came from residents, who themselves had been interns until the "day before yesterday." We saw the senior doctors on daily teaching rounds, and that was good, but when the sun went down over the Hudson River, we—the twenty-six- and twenty-eight-year-olds—were in charge. We knew the awesome responsibility that was on our shoulders, we cared deeply about the children who trusted us, and we were very much accountable to them. There was zero tolerance for mistakes of commission or omission, for failing to get lab results, for screwing up an IV placement. There would be hell to pay if you were responsible for an avoidable patient problem that was exposed during morning rounds with the chief resident or, far worse, the attending pediatrician.

We learned a lot. We worked all night in the ER treating children with severe asthma and raging fevers. We got very good at looking out into the waiting area and picking out the kid who was really sick and needed immediate attention. We staffed the newborn intensive unit, one of the most advanced in the nation at that time. That's where we learned—often from great nurses—how to get an IV line into a tiny scalp vein of a three-pound preemie.

All of us eventually experienced the pure exhilaration of resuscitating a child in extremis, how to quickly and effectively pass a breathing tube or do a lumbar puncture on a child being worked up for meningitis. But there were, as well, the experiences that gave us pause, the situations that made me, at least, question whether I had the fortitude to persist. I learned that, for whatever reason, I was inexorably drawn to the care of the sickest and most vulnerable children where every action mattered, every delay was potentially important, every wrong decision a possible disaster.

It wasn't always so rewarding. How could it be? There were moments when we had to deal with our own sheer panic and, perhaps a little too often, an emotional gut punch that made us feel helpless at a time and place where it seemed like some kind of action was needed, though we had no idea of what that might be.

Sometime during that first summer, I was called to the bedside of a two-year-old boy who had stopped breathing and lost his heartbeat thirty minutes earlier. My job was to "call" the baby—make the affirmative declaration that he was dead. Proximate causes of death were complications from a kidney cancer that didn't respond to chemotherapy, plus an infection that resisted whatever antibiotics we had available. The baby's body, still warm, looked very small on the big bed where he was being treated, and I wondered why he wasn't in a crib. From the window I could see Broadway, bustling with traffic and pedestrians. A woman's purse was on the tattered faux-leather armchair by the bed, probably the mother's, I thought. The only other person present was the floor nurse, Marie, busy trying to remove the bandages and tape covering the IVs and the soft gauze that was used to restrain the baby.

I looked at Marie's face, streaked with tears. "What's wrong?" I asked. "Are you OK?" Marie was experienced and savvy. She had seen a lot of tragedy during her seven years working the wards. She responded without looking at me, her hands busy pulling tape off the baby's left arm. "I did something terrible," she replied, pointing to the child's right hand. She had been using her surgical scissors to cut through the tape that had secured an IV in the baby's hand, and had accidentally snipped off the tip of his pinky. The baby was already gone; this purely accidental misfortune was immeasurably less awful than what he had endured in his final hospitalization. Mom had been in the room and watched in horror, moaning. Other floor staff took her to the waiting area.

The sight of the severed finger was too much for the mother, too much for Marie—and for me, too. I was mortified, so sorry for Marie, and overwhelmed by all of it. The children, the families, the work, the responsibilities—utter exhaustion was visible in her face and body language, and for a moment I just stared at Marie. She looked at me with nothing more to say about the incident, just "Can you help me get this baby cleaned up?"

On June 30, 1970, the internship came to an end. It had been a rite of passage and a year of indelible experiences that changed everything about my self-perception—a confidence-boosting sojourn through twelve intense months of life, death, suffering, triumph, and human experience.

It just took a few years to realize that I could and should bring an intensive-care sense of urgency to meeting the health care needs of underserved children. This was a slow-motion epiphany of finally understanding that poverty and racial disparities directly affect risk and vulnerability of children, especially those with extreme health care needs.

More to the point, children can't wait long for complex adversities to be remedied. Children are a dynamic "work in progress." Developmental and cognitive landmarks are critical; appropriate sensory and emotional inputs must coincide with specific stages of brain growth. Delays in timely positive input, or experiencing traumas that interfere with normal brain growth, may have permanent consequences. Advocacy for proper nutrition, the elimination of health barriers to learning or development, and the avoidance of "ACEs"—adverse childhood experiences—is a right-now situation. For some children, far too many, it's now or never.

Heading to the Delta, with a Layover in Denver

As much as I liked New York and the heady rewards of working at Columbia, in July 1971 I was offered a position in the pediatric training program at the University of Colorado, one of the hottest residencies in the country at the time. A spot had opened in the program because one of the residents had been drafted and refused his nearly automatic deferment. The big attraction of the pediatric residency in Denver had a little to do with the romantic backdrop of the Rockies west of the hospital—and a lot to do with the department chairman, a legendary clinician-teacher by the name of C. Henry Kempe.

I remember Kempe as a balding, "big presence" man with thick glasses and an enormous, uninterpretable smile. We liked to assume that his enigmatic grin was an indication that the chief was somehow pleased, but we never knew. Kempe died in 1984 at age sixty-two, shockingly young, though to me, as a young resident, he always seemed "old."

Kempe was a brilliant pediatrician, a mentor, and a leader in his field. He was the personification of wisdom to the medical students and residents who pretty much worshipped the man. Among a host of groundbreaking accomplishments, Kempe and a colleague identified and spoke out about a terrible scourge that until then had been largely ignored: the silent epidemic of child abuse and neglect in America. In 1962 he published a journal article on what he called the "battered child syndrome," launching a new and enduring focus on a problem that affected the lives of millions of children. The epidemic persists to this day: according to the American Society for the Positive Care of Children, in 2016 some 6.6 million children were involved in reports of abuse and neglect.[1] Most of these cases are "cleared," but at least one million reports each year are verified cases of child maltreatment.

Kempe had a broader philosophy that was groundbreaking in 1971. Our agenda as pediatricians in training focused on learning about how to medically care for sick children, of course, but he insisted that we also had to know about the environment, the family, and the level of nurturing and safety in the home of every patient we cared for. According to Kempe, it was not only well within our purview to investigate these issues, but our professional obligation to do so. In other words, we were professionally and ethically obliged to look beyond the strictly biomedical paradigm. He taught by example, interacting with children and parents at the bedside, his questions insightful and caring, his body language reflecting concern and focus. We, his eager minions, absorbed and learned by observation day after day on rounds in the children's wards of this enormous medical center at the foot of the Rockies.

For me—and my cohort of doctors in training—Kempe's influence was indelible. The lessons he taught, didactically and by example, never left.

One morning I accompanied Kempe to the labor and delivery suite where he had been called by one of the nurses to see a young woman who had delivered an infant boy just two hours earlier. There were no problems with the delivery and relatively little pain reported, as the mother had received spinal anesthesia. But the nurse was worried because the new first time mother, Lillian, had been crying nonstop and refused to hold the baby.

Dr. Kempe and I walked over to the bedside. Just to the right of her bed, the newborn was asleep in a bassinet, beautiful and quiet, swaddled in a blue striped blanket. Kempe spoke softly, greeted the mother, introducing himself and me, and pulled up a chair next to the bed. As he did so, he put a comforting hand on the young woman's shoulder. Then there was silence for several long moments. Mom was crying softly, and when she looked up to make eye contact with Kempe, he spoke again.

"Lillian, I am so glad to meet you. I know this is a complicated time, but I can't help noticing how beautiful your new baby is. But I am here to talk to you, first of all. How are you doing?"

Calmly and quietly, Kempe's focus remained on the mother. How was your pregnancy? What is your neighborhood like? How did you get ready for the new baby? Who will be available to help you with the baby? In short order, sensing genuine interest and concern from the old, grandfatherly professor, Lillian opened up. She and the baby's father were not married, and the relationship was clearly less than stellar. To further complicate matters, the father had an eight-year-old son from another relationship. Her new baby reminded her of the eight-year-old *and* the baby's father—and not in a good way. Standing at the foot of the bed, I was transfixed, soaking in the ambience, mostly concentrating on Kempe's focus and compassion that was so obvious and authentic.

When we left the room and were far enough down the hallway to be out of earshot, Kempe explained the dynamics of what we had just experienced. He carefully explained that this was a very high-risk situation, with early evidence of real bonding challenges that would not likely be solved without professional intervention that would need to begin even before discharge from the hospital. Then, this mother—and her newborn—would need intense in-home follow-up. This was a major child abuse problem waiting to happen. Lillian needed help and guidance immediately. But *if* we made all of this happen, there was a fighting chance that this risky situation could be turned around.

Kempe and I stopped at the nurses' station and he laid out the plan, making sure that all the critical appointments and arrangements would be organized. I never found out what happened with Lillian and her new baby, but I never forgot how Henry Kempe showed me what compassion and caring looked like in the real world of medical practice.

In my career, a focus on the extent and horrendous impact of child maltreatment in all its forms would result in creating actual programs to identify and treat the victims and perpetrators of abuse. In 1974 in Miami, I started the first such program in Florida. A decade later, I helped create a greatly expanded program—actually a center in its own building—at the Montefiore Medical Center in the Bronx.

Looking back on my year in Denver, I realize that just observing Henry Kempe up close and personal was a unique opportunity to see a master mentor at work. Every resident and medical student who had the good fortune to be inspired by Kempe learned about caring for children and families in ways that could not be easily described in textbooks or pediatric journals.

In 1971, as my residency year in Denver was coming to an end, my next career move was taking shape, or at least options were available. It wasn't an easy decision. I was deeply interested in social justice and public health, but my experiences as an intern dealing with very sick children led me to apply for, and be accepted in, a particularly competitive pediatric cardiology fellowship program with Dr. Jim Nora, chief of that specialty division at the time and a nationally reputed guru in the field. I appreciated the offer, but felt ambivalence. My thinking—maybe my rationalization—was that, even if I was going to end up focusing on activism and social change, I would need hard-core, unassailable medical credentials and skills to be credible.

Yet I still felt that this cardiology path was not quite right. I shared my uneasiness with my closest friend and fellow pediatric resident, Mike Kappy. "Why aren't I more excited about this Nora fellowship?" He said, "You know why. Just isn't quite you. At least not *all* of you." I knew Michael had it right; still, it was unsettling to be in this state of uncertainty. I could only hope that something would spark a higher level of passion and excitement. I needed another adrenaline rush. But when? And from where?

Both questions were eventually answered in the doctors' dining room at Denver Children's Hospital. Just inside the cafeteria, a large cork bulletin board was randomly covered with notices about schedules, lectures, job postings, lost and found items, and more. One day in April of 1971, I found myself drawn to a particular poster on the board. It was a message from VISTA (Volunteers in Service to America), a program created as part of President Lyndon Johnson's War on Poverty. Johnson's domestic policy guru, Sargent Shriver, had created VISTA as the domestic counterpart to JFK's Peace Corps. If you wanted to "do good" here in the United States, you joined VISTA. For many young Americans, VISTA was a direct connection to the front lines in the fight for social justice.

The poster included a powerful black-and-white photograph of a doctor with a black bag walking down a country road, his back to the camera. In the distance were some broken-down shacks in

a cotton field, a looming, haunting destination for what I imagined to be a young doctor on a mission. I imagined I knew him:
a dedicated, smart guy who uprooted himself, disconnected from
the expected career path, and headed to an unfamiliar place where
he would meet challenges he never could have dreamed of.

I saw myself in this picture. I stood there, transfixed, getting the
clarification I needed as a twenty-six-year-old doctor struggling to
define myself. This was the beginning of a journey that, twisting
and turning, would last a lifetime.

The text of the poster described the difficult conditions in Lee
County, Arkansas, where the VISTA doctor would work—directly
with and for the mostly, but not entirely, black, impoverished citizens
of Lee County. Most important to me, though, this opportunity also
offered the powerfully seductive chance to *do something*, as a doctor,
that would help bring about meaningful change.

This was quite literally about a chance to treat hopelessness—an
irresistible chance to help people overcome poverty and exclusion.
But here's the clincher. In bold, black letters at the very bottom of
the poster, it said, "If you're not part of the solution, you're part
of the problem." Hell no, I thought. No way was I going to be part
of this problem.

Still, it was the high-tech academic cardiology fellowship that
loomed large in my immediate future—that is, until I met Olly
Neal in a godforsaken dirt-poor county in East Arkansas. Adios,
prestigious fellowship . . .

The Mississippi Delta: A Long Way from Brooklyn

The VISTA poster listed Olly Neal, the clinic's executive director, as the point of contact. I came back to the dining room after
the lunch rush of doctors and nurses had cleared. Feeling excited
and dimly badass, I removed the poster from the bulletin board,
folded it in quarters, and headed back to the residents' lounge.

That afternoon I called Olly and arranged a visit. The following week he met me at the airport in Memphis, Tennessee.

The ride into eastern Arkansas couldn't have more disorienting. Leaving the outskirts of Memphis in Olly's pickup, we got deeper and deeper into an utterly unfamiliar environment. We rode through small impoverished hamlets, the road carving through soy and cotton fields, past shacks with sagging roofs, broken appliances on collapsing wooden porches, and wrecked cars and pickups in front yards, seemingly doomed to stay forever perched on cinder blocks. Yet somehow the experience was strangely exhilarating. We weren't even halfway to Lee County when I had already made a decision to accept the job, if the offer was made. But how on earth would I explain this to my wife?

Olly was a man in a hurry, and the sixty-five-mile trip over country roads took less than an hour. That said, he was ever on the alert for state and local police. A six-foot-three-inch black man getting stopped for speeding in the rural South in the early 1970s was a situation that he needed to avoid at all costs. Still, I had the feeling that Olly would be ready to deal with whatever happened.

Olly, who was born and raised in Lee County, spoke at a Southern country accented pace—that is, loud, clear, and articulate—telling me about the region's economy and history and the local struggles as they related to the turmoil roiling across the rest of the country. He framed the situation in this tiny, isolated county in rural Arkansas as part and parcel of the larger social and political transformation occurring across America at the time. Olly spoke, too, about the Lee County Cooperative Clinic and local politics. Children and elders stared at us as we barreled down Route 61. As we got closer to Marianna, the Lee County seat, more and more people recognized Olly's truck; we were greeted with waves and smiles by most, but also by the scowling faces of brawny white guys in pickup trucks.

As we rode into Marianna, Olly slowed the truck to a crawl. I got the full tour. "That's one of the old GPs' offices that just took down its 'colored waiting room' sign," Olly tells me. "And there's the private school for whites only." Whites controlled what little "wealth" there was and most definitely held all the political power in Lee County. Blacks had a decrepit, underfunded public school for their children and broken-down houses that regularly burned down because they were heated with dangerous kerosene heaters and coal- or wood-burning stoves.

Olly was a rising force in the Delta. In 1968 he helped organize a coalition of local black churches and a few small community-based organizations to convince VISTA to fund a small, comprehensive medical clinic in Marianna. Lacy Kennedy, the town's black funeral director, donated the space for the new clinic—a small house adjacent to the funeral parlor itself.

Dan Blumenthal, the first medical leader of the Lee County Cooperative Clinic (LCCC), started the program well before the actual clinic facility was identified and renovated. Dan was famous for practicing "out of the trunk" of his Ford Mustang. How cool!

I was profoundly moved by this unforgettable foray into a world that was totally foreign to me. Going back to Denver that evening, I was already dreading having to inform Dr. Nora that I wouldn't be taking his cardiology fellowship. But I was heading to Arkansas, no matter what he said—and no matter how guilty I felt.

As anticipated, Nora was not pleased, and my fellow residents were flabbergasted. The fellowship was a much-sought-after position, and I was pulling out just a couple of months before it was supposed to begin. People who knew me were not exactly surprised, just mortified that I would leave Nora hanging. They were right—this was not a good thing to do, and I truly felt bad about it. Dr. Nora was highly distressed, and I couldn't blame him. But this Arkansas gig, the poster, Olly Neal, and the challenge of working in the Delta made for an impossibly irresistible draw. It wasn't exactly about Vietnam or the Kent State shootings or the Freedom Fighters, but it was in the moment of massive protest and change in

America. Nothing was going to stop me from doing my part, defining my own role in the larger struggles, hunkering down in the belly of the Southern, racially ripped, poverty-infested beast of a culture.

After my highly uncomfortable conversation with Nora, I had to let the chairman, Henry Kempe, know about my decision to give up the fellowship with Nora. I wasn't looking forward to that conversation either. My buddy Kappy was reassuring. "Don't underestimate the old man's ability to adapt to change, especially for the kind of decision you've made." Helpful support, I thought—but I was still dreading this conversation with the chief.

To my surprise—and my great relief—Kempe smiled and interrupted me as I fumbled through my apologies, my big mea culpa regarding leaving Nora and the cardiology program hanging.

"Dr. Redlener, I understand what you're doing, and I get why. You told Jim that you're sorry, but you had to take this Arkansas job. Now you can also tell him that I support your decision." Relieved, I hugged my old professor and mentor, thanking him profusely, but anxious to get out of his office.

A couple of months later, at the graduation ceremony for the residents, Kempe mentioned each of us, saying a little about our specific plans following training. Some of us were taking advanced subspecialty training (as I was supposed to), but the majority were headed to pediatric private practice. When he got to me, Kempe said, "Most of you are going to private practice—and that's great. But our own Dr. Redlener is heading to rural Arkansas to run a VISTA clinic, and there, amidst poverty and turmoil, Irwin will be doing 'public' practice." Yes, indeed.

My immediate predecessor running the LCCC was Dr. Robbie Wolf, Dan Blumenthal's successor. Robbie was an indefatigable optimist in a strange and very difficult environment. He was one of the most extraordinarily dedicated physicians I have ever met—before or since. Just before I arrived to take his place, I received a twelve-page, single-spaced typed letter from Robbie. In exquisite detail, he explained the clinic's routine and described those who would sustain and support me—as well as need my help—over the next extraordinary two years. Among the "cast of characters" on Robbie's seventy-person list were Olly and other clinic staff; Olly's brother, Prentiss, a member of Concerned Citizens of Lee Country, a black political organization; clinic landlord Lacy Kennedy; black preachers; some desperately poor patients; and Ruth Prestridge, a "rich white lady and potential friend." I didn't know at the time how much of a friend Ruth would turn out to be.

Robbie also warned me about the political and racial climate I was walking into. Blacks had received such disrespectful treatment when seeking medical care elsewhere in Lee County in the past "that they would rather stay home and die than get treated rudely or unfeelingly anymore," he wrote. Given this history, and the general lack of transportation among the poor, Robbie made a lot of house calls, and he advised me to do the same.

From Robbie's letter:

Right now most patients come to us by word of mouth, from friends who are our patients who dig our service. People come in large numbers for three reasons:

1. *We are free*
2. *We get a lot of cures*
3. *We are kindly*

None of these things are good enough by themselves to keep the patients coming back; all three are crucial, the first because the folks have no bread [money], the second because a lot of people here don't believe in doctors because they are unconvinced by . . . past [experiences] that docs can do much more than cure pneumonia, the third because poor people in general, and blacks in particular, in the county have received disrespectful first name treatment by office help for [too] long. . . . If you gear the whole operation with the three little maxims in mind that I just mentioned, you can't lose and you'll have more patients than you'll know what to do with, which is currently the case.

Robbie's letter also described the deteriorating relationship between the clinic and the twenty-five-bed Lee County Hospital—a totally inadequate medical facility if ever I saw one, but the only hospital in the county. In essence, the hospital was desperately trying to deny admission privileges to the LCCC doctors. Denial of admitting privileges for our physicians based on some trumped up violation of a procedural formality was a real hardship; it meant that we had to admit our sick patients to a larger facility in Helena, Arkansas, more than twenty-six miles away.

The situation was incredibly inconvenient for the medical staff, taking us too far, for too many hours every day, from the high-risk community we were serving. Even more concerning, being hospitalized so far from Lee County was an intolerable burden for our patients and their families. Public transportation was essentially nonexistent, and many people in the county didn't have a working car. Furthermore, Helena, with its population of 10,000, was a big, unfamiliar "city" to some people in Lee County. Many poor, black residents of the county had spent their entire lives without traveling more than fifteen miles from their homes. The hospital in Helena, and the travails of just getting there, seemed more than a little foreboding to them. I could only imagine.

I was deeply moved by Robbie's words, drawn even more to Lee County, still a mysterious and foreign place where I would have to find a way to do what needed to be done in an environment still frozen in the poverty, racism, and disparities of the "Old South." Although I never spent more than a few hours with Robbie in person, his authenticity, his compassion, and that beautiful letter made me always think of this doctor, hardly two years older than I was, as one of my most significant mentors.

Arlene and I, with our two children in tow, arrived in Marianna in early July and found a rental house within walking distance of the Lee County Cooperative Clinic. The clinic itself was in a minimally renovated house on the property of the only black-owned funeral parlor in the county. Lacy Kennedy, the owner of the establishment and the clinic's landlord, was reputed to be one of the few blacks in Lee County who "had money."

By the time we arrived in Lee County, I had been married to Arlene for six years. Our two children, four-year-old David and one-year-old Jason, would be involuntary transplants to the rural South, never questioning how or why they got to a tattered rental house a couple of blocks from the Lee County Cooperative Clinic in Marianna, Arkansas.

David was enrolled in a local Head Start preschool program with mostly poor black kids (and a few very poor white kids with horrendously bad teeth). He was happy, which was more than I can say for the family next door to us. They regularly tossed rocks into our backyard, yelling "nigger lovers." Charming. I was too naïve to realize how dangerous this county could be for a carpetbagging New York doctor who was there explicitly to care for the marginalized and impoverished black population who were forever the second-class citizens of East Arkansas.

Besides those nasty but basically trivial incidents in the backyard, I was dealing with a host of serious threats, subtle and otherwise. The white population of the county despised the clinic and its organizers—especially Olly Neal. Then, too, I was particularly loathed as an outspoken, aggressive, long-haired, northern Jew. I was followed regularly by members of the White Citizens' Council—angry, glaring men with rifles in the gun racks fixed to the back windows of their pickup trucks.

Just to be sure we got the message, one night Arlene and I were awoken just before 1:00 a.m. by the sounds of gunning engines and screeching tires. We ran to the window and saw a crude, three-foot-high wooden cross burning on the front lawn. I tried to call Olly—no answer. I knew the sheriff would be uninterested, at best, in hearing from me; at worst, he might be among the cross-burners. Getting back to sleep was tough, and the next days were nerve-wracking. Every white person looked suspicious to me. Was *that* guy at my house last night?

Still I was unstoppable and determined to make a difference—medically and politically—in Lee County. That intensity, that fervor, may have been one of the reasons my marriage was getting shakier by the month as we tried to make it in Lee County. It was clear to me that this lifestyle wasn't what Arlene had bargained for—not the suburban practice and lifestyle that she had in mind when, at ages twenty-one and twenty respectively, we got married in a synagogue in the upper-middle-class community of Woodmere, Long Island, just twenty-five miles due east of Manhattan. We tried to make it work in the Delta, but it was tough. The stress was high and persistent, in large part due to my intense focus on the mission and the strange exhilaration that came from working somewhere that mattered, where it would make a difference. This was a health care challenge, to be sure, but it was also a struggle for social justice—everything else be damned.

Had I fallen overboard, drifting away from my family, a bit intoxicated with self-righteousness? Maybe. But this was a strange place, and Arlene wasn't in the center of the action and the energy. I was the self-proclaimed world-changer; Arlene, misjudged or not, was a bystander, seemingly content as a housewife and mother.

What was the breaking point? Maybe that afternoon when Arlene was in our backyard and happened to notice a couple of children next door by the side of the house where a particularly unwelcoming, unpleasant white family lived. The twelve-year-old boy, pants around his ankles, was standing behind his whimpering six-year-old sister, pressing against her. "Stand still!" he barked. She cried. Arlene yelled, "Stop it! What are you doing?" The boy picked up his pants; his sister, naked from the waist down, looked terrified. Not knowing what to do, Arlene ran next door. The children's young mother seemed barely interested. "Boys will be boys," she said. Arlene was aghast—if she ever needed more evidence that there was no way she would ever adapt to living in Lee County, this was it.

Eventually, before the end of our first year in Lee County, we separated. Arlene moved to Miami, Florida, taking David and Jason with her. This was tough to bear. I had no idea how to resolve the emotional turmoil of guilt, obligation, loyalty, and a profoundly important connection to my boys. The situation was basically a mess—and I dealt with it by immersing myself in the work, distracted constantly by the challenges of practicing in this run-down, depressing throwback to a very bad time in the American South, which in 1972, my second year in the county, was still steeped in poverty and racism.

Practicing at the clinic was a daily adventure of unpredictable situations and challenges. Within a month of being in the county, a baby who had been born at home—in a shack in the western part of the county—was brought in to see me, carried by his father in a badly stained, torn cardboard box. Swathed in a dirty blanket, crying and hungry, the infant, an emaciated older sibling, and their forlorn mother conveyed everything I needed to know about practicing pediatrics in America's sixth poorest county.

The VISTA volunteers assigned to the Lee County Cooperative Clinic were extraordinary individuals, each one of them. But there was one in particular who would change everything for me about being in East Arkansas and understanding what was possible for the children of Lee County.

Soon after I arrived, it became apparent that many children in the county were developmentally delayed and needed to be evaluated for possible referral to appropriate intervention programs. (There were no such programs—yet—in Lee County, but we had to start somewhere.) I asked Olly to request a social worker volunteer from the national VISTA pool that was being oriented and trained in Houston.

Olly called the regional office and told them to expect a formal request for a social worker. Unfortunately, no one with such a skill set was available. What they could do, however, was send us a young, recent graduate of Pomona College in Los Angeles.

She was not a social worker—but she had majored in *sociology*. Close enough for government work.

The story ended well—much better than we anticipated. Karen Blomberg arrived at the clinic a few weeks later. She was more than eager to get into the ebb and flow of our mission. She was beautiful, aggressively independent, used to doing her own thing, a dedicated progressive from a family of intensely conservative Republicans. Karen had volunteered in Head Start programs while she was still in college and was ready to take on this new job.

We trained her to do comprehensive health screening for children throughout the county. In fact, to help provide the expertise she would need to do child developmental assessment, I sent her to Denver to work with some of the professionals I had met as a resident. Karen ultimately screened nearly a thousand children for developmental delays and established some very innovative intervention programs. And she pushed hard to do more, training local staff, establishing social services, and developing community support programs.

Karen's work with me and for the children of Lee County inexorably generated the kind of mysterious vibe that ultimately emerged as a crazy kind of romance, perhaps not uncommon in the intense atmosphere of full-on commitment to a vital mission, especially one with overtones of tension and danger. By the time I was ready to leave Arkansas at the end of my two-year contract, it was abundantly clear to me that I wouldn't be going anywhere without Karen.

Among the most important and endearing experiences in Lee County were the daily house calls. Every evening, after clinic hours, I visited poor sick people living in the outer reaches of Lee County where there was no available public transportation. Even if there had been a convenient way to make the trek, these folks were often too ill to make it to my clinic. What about an ambulance to the Lee County Hospital? That was out of the question. The single ambulance in the county was rarely available, especially for poor black families who could never pay for such services.

So I would head to their homes, where I would sit at the bedsides, grateful family members thanking me for coming to see grandpa with a recent stroke or the dehydrated toddler with incessant diarrhea. I did what I could, sometimes starting an IV right there in the dark living room, sometimes leaving medications, and occasionally making arrangements for an urgent trip to the emergency room of a major hospital in Little Rock or Memphis. But most of all, the house calls were unparalleled opportunities to meet and get to know the families we were there to care for. It was in those intimate encounters that the community learned to trust us, and where we could see and absorb what it meant to live with adversities that were part and parcel of living amid profound rural poverty.

It was all thrilling—hard-core medical practice *and* a chance to make a profound difference in a community where it really mattered. Looking back, Lee County in the early 1970s was one of the only places I've been where most—though never all—children did not nurture aspirations, learning early that surviving, not dreaming, was their mission, just as it was for their parents and grandparents.

The people who joined the staff at the clinic created a special culture that added much to my own experience there. About half of the team was composed of locals, many born and raised in Lee County. We identified highly motivated people anxious to learn the skills and do the jobs we needed in the clinic. We sent them for training or trained them ourselves. The rest of the crew consisted of VISTA volunteers who came from everywhere to play their part in the struggle to make America better, to heal communities.

One of the most poignant memories I have is that in spite of the challenges, the danger, and the recurrent moments of hopelessness, I was still oddly, ironically optimistic. Sincere and perhaps irrationally certain, I told anyone who would listen that the conditions of deprivation, injustice, and severe economic disparities would soon be over. My frequently articulated prediction was that in a decade, maybe fifteen years, change would be manifest. Poverty would be ended, and every child would have access to good health care and a decent school. It was simply unimaginable that what we saw in Arkansas could possibly last. I never could have—or would have—predicted that the child poverty rate would still be over 20 percent more than four decades later, or that children would still be having severe problems accessing medical care, or that more than half of the youth in some poor communities across the United States would not graduate from high school on time.

Adapting to life in Lee County was a two-way street. For sure, I had to adapt to an unusual and unfamiliar environment, but I was also very aware that, one way or another, we had to be accepted by the people we were serving—a goal more easily achieved than I had imagined. The fact is that we just loved being there, helping people who trusted us to care for them, and I think that was apparent to our patients and their families. Condescension toward our patients was not acceptable. We were a team of highly qualified professionals, but authentic human beings fiercely committed to the community we served without pretension. My predecessor, Robby Wolf, had advised me to "be kind," but that was hardly a message that any of us needed to hear. To a person, workers from the community and volunteers from everywhere else all shared a commitment to the well-being of the patients and families who had brought us together in the first place.

Life as a doctor in Lee County was a constant feast of immersion in the community and in our work. The clinic was always packed with people desperate for care, people with conditions caused or exacerbated by what are known as the "social determinants" of health. Poverty, poor sanitation, and nutritional inadequacy contributed to the sky-high rates of hypertension, heart disease and stroke, pediatric diarrhea, and stunted growth.

Children would appear in the clinic with gross malnutrition or diseases like mumps or measles that should have been eradicated by immunizations—if primary care had been reliably available before we arrived in the community. Many children had apparent developmental delays or hearing loss from untreated or poorly treated ear infections. More than once I cared for newborns born "back at the house," brought in to see me for their first checkups. Families did not have and could not afford bassinets, car carriers, strollers, or carriages.

And then there was the constant need to be "medical detectives," though now we would characterize that as being experts in solving public health challenges. For instance, our medical teams would see very sick children coming for care of persistent watery diarrhea and dehydration. We would treat them with antibiotics, fluids, and medicines to control diarrhea. Sometimes they required hospitalization for intravenous fluids. Then, a month or two later, they would be back again with the same symptoms. This was the recurring pattern of care until one day at an all-staff meeting, Harry Conard, a trained sanitation engineer who was serving as a VISTA volunteer, had a brilliant insight.

"You know what, guys," he started, "I've been thinking about this recurrent diarrhea situation. So I went and visited some of the communities where this is particularly bad and saw that many of these houses had privies built way too close to the water pump. We're probably just getting recurrent contamination of the drinking water."

Harry was right, of course. So the community treatment plan was straightforward: our staff, working with some volunteer med students visiting from Boston and members of the local communities, spent about six weeks helping many families build new privies, this time safely distant from the water pumps. Problem solved!

What about the fact that so many of our patients were being injured, sometimes even killed, by home fires? And children being burned on wood-burning stoves? Here again, a broader look, outside traditional medical tools, would be necessary.

Arkansas is not in the tropics. On a winter evening it can get downright chilly, but many of our patients lived in rickety shacks without central heat. To make do, families had small wood- or kerosene-burning stoves, tempting targets for crawling babies and mobile toddlers. A bigger problem was that the kerosene heater was often placed directly under the window to help neutralize the chill coming from outside. Time after time, house fires would start from a dangling curtain, ignited by the stove or heater. Our solution was to inform patients about our concerns and suggest moving the heater a safer distance away from the window. That's about all we could do.

We made the daily house calls, and we drove patients to see specialists in Little Rock and Memphis. We stood up for them and fought to make sure they got the care they needed. More than that, we talked as equals; we laughed and cried together. We had dinner in their homes and ate things like chitterlings (known as "chitlins")—a horrifying sausage-like concoction of pigs' intestines and whatever spices might be available.

A family we got to know well were the Patricks. Evelyn and Walter had four children, two of whom were sick with a variety of chronic illnesses, including the now very rare condition known as rheumatic fever (RF). In the pre-antibiotic era, RF was a major scourge of childhood, a complication of the common strep throat that, left untreated, could cause severe heart disease, arthritis, and other secondary conditions. Once the antibiotic penicillin was widely introduced into medical practice in the 1940s, the incidence of diseases like RF dropped dramatically. In fact, until I met Sherry Patrick, then just ten years old, I had never seen a case of this disease, only read about it. Penicillin had essentially eradicated RF, except for the occasional outbreak in highly impoverished communities where access to doctors—and antibiotics—was far from assured.

In the fall of 1972, Walter sent me an urgent message. "Doctor Redlener, Walter Patrick called," said Cora, the nurse assistant.

"He wants you to come out and help him. He said it was an emergency."

Cora was a total gem, a friendly African American woman and third-generation resident of Marianna. She was one of the locals trained by our program staff to become a nursing assistant. She was beloved in the community and by her colleagues in the clinic. More than that, she was one of the people who helped me get oriented and comfortable in Lee County.

"Sure," I responded. "Is it one of the kids?"—fully expecting to hear something worrisome about Sherry or one of the babies.

"Not really. Nobody from the family."

"Then what? A neighbor?" Cora leaned over my desk and made very direct eye contact, a big smile on her face.

"Actually," she continued, "he says that his *hog* has a problem. Seems to be in pain, and old Walter thinks he sees a 'rupture.'"

"You mean a hernia?"

"That's what I think he's talking about."

I had already been in Arkansas for a year, so not much would really surprise me. But a hog with a hernia was way, way beyond what I could have possibly expected.

"What do I know about hog hernias? I'm a pediatrician, not a veterinarian! And besides, surgery was not exactly my best subject in med school."

Cora smiled at me. "Doc, you know very well that there isn't a vet within thirty miles of here. And anyway, nobody will go out to their farm. They're a truly dirt-poor black family. It's you or nobody."

I sat there thinking about Walter, his family, this godforsaken county, and the sick hog. I just shook my head and kind of smiled at Cora.

"Up you go," she said. "I'll get your bag and some surgical tools."

"Fine. And don't forget some injectable tranquilizers and Novocain."

The important thing about that hog was that the Patricks were raising the animal to sell at the market, bringing some badly needed money to the family. This animal, in other words, was a key part of the family's livelihood and its immediate future.

I asked Karen Blomberg to join me.

"You sure you want *me* to go?" (The truth was I *always* wanted her to go.)

"Absolutely," I answered. "And bring the video camera."

The Patricks' farm was in Turkey Scratch, about twenty miles from the clinic. We took the clinic's old, yellow-painted U.S. Army surplus Jeep that had been acquired the year before in a government auction. The drive out of town included a lot of laughs about this bizarre experience we were about to have, mixed with a good dose of anxiety and a serious discussion of what was at stake for our friends and patients, the Patrick family.

We drove up the dirt one-lane road leading up to the Patricks' house and spotted Walter and the older kids standing by the pen just in front of their small barn. Evelyn was up by the house, holding the baby, Annie. She waved and smiled, and we waved back, but we pulled up near Walter. He was decidedly *not* smiling and looked clearly distressed as he came over to open the Jeep's door.

"I'm so glad you here, Doc. We're real worried about this hog. I think she's got a rupture."

"Look, Walter," I said, "you know I would do anything for you, but I don't do surgery, really. And I have never, ever treated any animal—particularly a pig!"

"I figured that. But I appreciate you coming here. I tried to get a vet, but it weren't going to happen."

I sighed and got out of the car. Karen was right behind. "Let's take a look."

"Karen, make sure, at least, that you capture this craziness on the video. I have a feeling that I might have to prove this whole thing actually happened to somebody at some point."

Karen smiled, and with Walter leading the way, off we went into the pen. The sow was lying there in the corner, breathing what seemed to be very rapidly—though, truth be told, I had no idea of the "normal" respiratory rate of a two-year-old hog. "Walter, is this hog breathing faster than normal?"

"Oh, yeah. And she feels really hot to me."

As I approached the animal, she kept a wary eye on me, but stayed still. She was lying on her side, and it didn't take a physical examination to see the enormous bulge on her lower abdomen. I put on a pair of rubber gloves and very slowly, very gently, palpated the tense mass, but there was something about the bulge, the lethargy, and what Walter seemed to indicate might be a fever.

"This might be an abscess," I say to Walter. "Let's try to drain it."

Now I was worried. This hog was sick, too sick to eat or sell, but in my personal "fog of war" at that moment, I decided that I needed to do something—at least *try*, for the family's sake. I got out the kit Cora had prepared and loaded up one syringe with Novocain and a second with whatever tranquilizer she had packed. Prepping the area with disinfectant, I injected the furry skin over the mass with a syringe full of anesthetic. The hog snorted and tried to stand up. Walter was, more or less, holding her in place. My plan was to give the animal a whopping dose of tranquilizer and at least try to drain the apparent abscess.

After waiting a few slow-moving minutes for the Novocain to set in, I injected the medicine into the muscular area on the back of her hind leg. Now she was moving a lot more, and Walter was having trouble holding her still.

"Hey, Evelyn, come on over here and give us a hand!" Walter yelled out.

Evelyn handed the baby to Sherry, ran into the pen, and wrapped her strong arms around the animal's head. It was time for me to act. Using a scalpel, I pierced the bulging mass, and two things happened in rapid succession. First a huge amount of yellow-green pus began flowing out of the incision I had just made. (Abscess confirmed!) Then the hog broke loose from Walter and Evelyn and, with some horrifying hog screaming, proceeded to bolt around the pen, repeatedly bumping into the fence and attempting to leap in the air.

Karen was frozen in disbelief and fear. She had captured most of the "surgery" and now was just standing there with the camera pointing to the ground.

"Karen, keep on filming!"

Eventually we got control of the exhausted and feverish hog, and I had to break the news to the farmer and his wife.

"So sorry." The hog was too sick, and was dying from a terrible infection.

"I understand. And thanks for trying." Walter said, his eyes tearing.

"We appreciate all you do," added Evelyn.

Karen and I went up to the rickety porch of the family's house and spent a few minutes with the children, especially with my patient Sherry, who wasn't looking that great. I said she needed to come into Marianna and get checked. That was the plan for tomorrow, she assured me.

Karen and I got back in the car and were driving back toward the highway when we heard a gunshot, probably the twelve-gauge Walter owned. As we learned the next day when Evelyn brought her daughter to see me in the clinic, that's how the hog was put out of its misery, at the same time making the Patricks' financial situation even more uncertain than it usually was.

Olly Neal

There were many incredible people in Lee County, but none more powerful or inspiring than Olly Neal. I was in awe watching his ability to articulate positions, to deal with people from all walks of life; he was nuanced and effective in ways I have rarely seen, before or since. Olly seemed to be above the idea of holding a grudge, even with those I would see as morally reprehensible, political mortal enemies. There were lots of very bad people in the county, but Olly was far smarter than I was about all of this. In the real-world process of breaking down color walls, he was a lot more successful, too.

As I settled into life in Lee County, getting to know Olly and watching him in action, I came to see him as the anchor of this health care experiment, though far more than that. He was the force and the cover story—and I was along for the ride, fully engaged and in the tumultuous mix before I even unpacked our boxes.

Every once in a while, Olly would get angry, his expression fixed, gaze unwavering, language direct. When he wasn't intense, he was relaxed and extraordinarily sociable and funny—a storyteller supreme. Still, even in those moments of easygoing levity, he looked as though he could erupt at any moment. You really wouldn't want to be the target of his wrath.

Olly projected a larger-than-life and unique charisma. He was revered by the black community, but he scared many—though not all—of the white minority who, in the early 1970s, still held the political and financial power in Lee County. When it came to Olly Neal, there was always the sense of volatility and some ill-defined danger for those who would, overtly or covertly, dare to express or promote injustice or racism. Though Olly's anger was mostly controlled, it would periodically be on display, purposefully for the effect it had on people and perhaps, too, for the sheer drama of confrontation.

Olly had a chameleonic capacity to adapt to his surroundings. His powerful voice could easily dominate negotiations, and often did, but he could also retreat to a kind of Southern demeanor of compromise when he needed to. He would speak in the authentic dialect of a rural black man when we were in Marianna or visiting a family in some remote outpost of the county, but when called for, his persona—and diction—would seamlessly morph into that of an urbane, educated man articulating a position or a highly quotable, inscrutable source for the *Commercial Appeal*, a great newspaper out of Memphis. That's how he was with visiting academics and the many politicians he met in Little Rock and Washington, DC—no rabid troublemaker, just a powerful, fearless man on a mission, making a case, understanding the big picture, the history and societal dynamics of the great turmoil playing out in his county.

Olly had federal agencies in the Department of Health, Education, and Welfare practically swooning over starting new programs in the Delta—at least until much of this activity was stopped by President Richard Nixon's hatchet man, Howard Phillips. Nixon appointed Phillips as director of the Office of Economic Opportunity (OEO) with the expressed purpose of dismantling that agency, created under Lyndon Johnson's War on Poverty.

Always "the boss," Olly was a master of managing relationships with people who started out hostile but, in some weird, counterintuitive way, ended up friends with the charismatic community leader. He was supremely skilled at breaking down color barriers and preconceived, race-based misperceptions that had been held for generations.

Just prior to my arrival in Lee County, the slow burn of racial tension sparked into a dangerous firestorm. A young black girl ordered a slice of pizza in a tiny, white-owned restaurant on Marianna's town square. After enduring a slew of inappropriate and racist comments, the girl walked out—without her pizza. The man behind the counter called the sheriff, who promptly arrested the girl for "breach of contract" because she did not buy the food she ordered. That incident ignited a tinderbox. Fire bombings, a black boycott of white businesses in Marianna, and the threat of explosive violence pushed then governor Dale Bumpers to assert state control over the county and its 18,000 citizens. Within hours of the first call to the governor's office, Bumpers assigned about forty Arkansas National Guard troops to enforce a nighttime curfew in Lee County.

As a physician, I was permitted to be on the streets during the curfew. After all, I had house calls to make and patients to see in the local hospital.

I had a call from Olly Neal, who, of course, was granted no such curfew exemption. It was a particularly humid night in late July, and Olly had received a call from our clinic administrator, Alice Morganfield, who told him that her house was being threatened, presumably by armed men associated with the Klan or the White Citizens' Council. So Olly called me asking if I would drive him to Alice's place.

I got to Olly's house as quickly as I could. It was unbearably hot, so I was a shocked to see him wearing an overcoat, carrying a briefcase. "What's up, Olly?" He said nothing, got in the car, and opened his coat, revealing a pump-action shotgun. I learned later that his briefcase was filled with ammunition. Mr. Neal was preparing for war. Fifteen minutes later, we were at Alice's house in Aubrey, Arkansas, a tiny village—population 350—some twelve miles southwest of Marianna.

The house was on the one gravel road in town, and with a cloud cover obscuring the moonlight, it was difficult for me to tell how close she was to any neighbors. Alice's car was parked near the house, and a pickup truck was stationed on the front lawn. It had arrived a bit before Olly and I did, having transported a few of Alice's friends, also ready for action if the need arose. There was no denying my sense of fear and foreboding—but inexplicable exhilaration, too. I probably would have just stayed with everyone else in the truck or in Alice's house waiting for something to happen, but Olly had a very clear idea of what needed to happen. Getting out of the car, he turned back to me, "Get out of here. Now!"

I wanted to stay. I was pumped, ready for who knows what, but this was not up for debate.

The upshot? I did what Olly wanted and got the hell home!

Only the next morning did I learn that the shooters never materialized or ran off, and Alice, Olly, and the rest were, thankfully, unharmed.

Death and Misunderstanding

The jaw-dropping experiences while living in that sleepy yet deeply seething Southern town desperately trying to hold onto a dying past never seemed to end. My friend from Denver, Mike Kappy, visited in November of 1971, just a few months after I arrived in the county. We had totally bonded during residency and determined to stay in touch, but it was his idea to actually come to Lee County. For one thing, he was curious about this strange place and wanted to see it for himself. He never exactly said so, but I think he was worried about me, too. He kept telling me it wasn't actually safe for me, especially knowing how aggressive and outspoken I was.

In addition to being one of the smartest pediatricians I had ever met, Michael had other talents, including high-end furniture making—though I never really understood how he acquired that skill. He was also a talented photographer, and during his visit he took a gallery's worth of beautiful and compelling pictures of the children and families whose struggles had brought me to Lee County in the first place. Then, because our friends and patients the Lotts had no place for their newest baby to sleep other than the parents' bed, already occupied every night by the two of them and one of the older children, Michael built them a beautiful rocking cradle.

Perhaps to reinforce Michael's concerns for my safety in the county, one afternoon we had an unusual reception by storekeepers along one of the ramshackle streets in Marianna's town square, just down the block from the Lee County Courthouse, the seat of power. As we walked toward the gazebo in the center of the square, one after another, shopkeepers came out of their stores to stare at us. Each held a baseball bat in one hand and slapped the palm of the other hand with the barrel of the bat. Michael was shaken. I was just pissed.

Most days at the clinic more or less fell into a routine, but that never lasted more than a week. In early 1972, I was on call for the hospital and got a frantic message that there had been a terrible wreck on the highway. Unfortunately, there was no other physician in the county that afternoon. I raced to the hospital's little emergency area and saw a woman on a blood-splattered gurney, literally dying before my eyes. Her husband was waiting in the hallway, and I closed the exam room door. She had a massive head injury and was barely breathing. The nurse was attempting to help her breathe with an Ambu bag and oxygen. A pulse monitor showed a slow, irregular heartbeat. And she was very pregnant—in her eighth month, according to the nurse.

I asked for a stethoscope and examined her abdomen, hearing the faint heartbeat of the baby, apparently still alive. It was a moment of truth. I had trained as a pediatrician and had been at many cesarean sections when there was trouble anticipated for the newborn, but I had never done a C-section myself.

There was zero time to ponder a course of action here. I decided to try to save the baby and asked the nurse to open a surgical kit. We rapidly draped the mother's abdomen and prepped the area with an iodine solution. I know I was sweating, but didn't have the luxury of hesitating. I cut through the skin, through the abdominal wall, and into the uterus.

"Doc, we lost her pulse and her color is bad."

"Yes," I responded, "she's gone. But I am going to try to save this baby."

In the background I heard her husband yelling, "Where's Linda? How is she? How's our baby? Don't let them die!"

He had not been in the pickup truck his wife was driving. Another car, apparently driven at high speed by a very intoxicated teenager from a local farm family, crossed the dividing line and hit the pickup head on. The teenager had died instantly.

Arkansas troopers were with my patient's husband on the other side of the door, trying to keep him calm, though how would that even be possible? Meanwhile I was determined to do everything I could to at least save that baby.

As soon as I extracted the infant boy from the womb, I knew this was not going to end well. Even deep inside the protection of the uterus, the amniotic fluid, and the mother's abdomen, the force of the impact had caused serious and visible injuries to the baby. I heard no more heartbeat. Resuscitation would be to no avail. I stood there by the gurney trying to calm myself and process what had just happened. The nurse, looking like she was in shock, was tending to the mother. I was holding the dead infant and, after a long minute or two, passed him to the aide.

Now I knew that I had to do something that I could not possibly be dreading more. I needed to go out and speak with the husband who had just lost his wife and his baby.

I walked through the door and saw him, a bruiser of a guy, maybe six feet two or three inches. He had a straggly beard and a John Deere hat, face flushed and teary.

"How is she, doc? And how's our baby?"

I leaned over to him and whispered, "We tried, but they didn't make it."

It must have been my muffled voice and my northern accent, but it still stands out as one of the most horrific experiences of my career—indeed, of my life. Whatever the explanation—maybe it was just the consequence of wishful thinking—the guy thought I said something like "She's alive; they're going to make it."

Now he was sobbing, embraced me with two huge arms, "Oh thank Jesus, doc. Thank you, thank you . . . thank you, Jesus." I was frozen, clearly in some form of emotional shock myself, now evolving into plain fear. What the hell was I supposed to do now?

I backed out of his grip and saw the trooper a few feet from us, just trying to absorb this whole scene.

"No, no, sir. I am so sorry. I said, 'They didn't make it.' They didn't make it, either one of them."

The man's eyes widened, he was beyond incredulous, and after a few seconds of absorbing the reality of the situation, he screamed at me—first a guttural, primal sound, then charging toward me, yelling "What? What? You let them die? I'm going to kill you!" If that Arkansas State Police officer and a male hospital aide hadn't been able to wrestle that very distraught, big angry man to the ground, he just might have actually killed me, right there in the hallway of the Lee County Memorial Hospital.

Joan Baez: The Madonna Meets Marianna

There was no end to the crazy and surreal packed into those two years in Arkansas. I was isolated, though never alone. I was living in the ultimate godforsaken town of old cotton plantations and soybean fields, with no real restaurants to speak of and not a movie theater in the county. There were some white folks and a few blacks who lived in relative affluence, including the Prestridge family, who owned a cotton gin and lived in a neat brick house in one of Marianna's white enclaves. Then there were the Daggetts, a prominent white Lee County family who had lived in the region for generations. Young Jesse Daggett, a friend of Olly Neal for years, was an attorney; he and Ruth Prestridge were probably the only two white citizens who were actually friendly to us. Ruth had met my predecessor, the inimitable Dr. Robbie Wolfe, and they had become real friends.

Jesse and Ruth didn't always agree with us, but they were very helpful, concerned for us personally, sympathetic to what we were doing, and supportive of our efforts to bring good medical care to the impoverished black families of Lee County.

Jesse did the best he could to advise the team through some of the complex political situations that plagued the clinic on a regular basis. When the local hospital tried to exclude our VISTA doctors from getting admitting privileges, a real hardship for the medical team—and the thousands of people we were trying to care for—Jesse was guiding us from behind the scenes. This was never a straightforward question of meeting the admitting privilege "standards" of a primitive, twenty-five-bed facility in southeastern Arkansas. This was, like almost every issue in the Delta, a question of white control, deep resentment of the northern interlopers with white coats and stethoscopes, and a relentless clinging to the values and traditions of a starkly segregated community struggling with the slow-moving, inevitable social change that was destined to fundamentally reshape the culture—and politics—of the deep South.

Ruth Prestridge's husband, Albert, was hard to read and, we all suspected, not very supportive of Ruth's admiration for Olly Neal, the VISTA team, and me. The first time Ruth introduced me to "good ol' boy" Al was a little stressful.

"Hi, Mr. Prestridge, good to meet you."

He glared at me, taking full measure of this young, long-haired, mustachioed, hippie, Jewish doctor from New York City—who, I am sure he was convinced, was out to destroy his way of life.

"Likewise," said a decidedly unsmiling Mr. Albert Emerson Prestridge. That was the whole, unvarnished conversation; the awkward silence was broken by an astute Ruth inviting us to enjoy a glass of Southern tea.

Throughout our stint in Arkansas, Ruth was kind to all of us and inexplicably receptive to whatever we requested. I suspected that underneath the veneer, and in spite of Al's disapproval, his doting wife just basically was not comfortable with the overt racism in Lee County. She had sincere sympathy for the plight of the indigent black community and was happy to help the upstarts make sure that everyone in her community got the care they needed. And it was a two-way street.

One day I received a call that Ruth and Al's son was in trouble. After an alcohol binge, the teenager was found comatose in a field just outside of town. I got there as soon as I could and found a young man in serious medical trouble—rapid heart rate, very shallow breathing, cool to the touch, and unresponsive. We got him stabilized with nasal oxygen, warm blankets, and an IV. It being a decade and half before cell phones would be available, I sent somebody to bring an ambulance, which arrived twenty minutes later, and we got young Prestridge to the medical center in Memphis. He would be fine, but, as they say, it could have been a lot worse.

Ruth was always fond of us, but after we came to the aid of her son, we were bonded in ways that went beyond her connection to the mission that inspired our work in Lee County. She was vested in the very idea of the Lee County Cooperative Clinic and deeply grateful to our team. So when Joan Baez, the legendary folk singer—often referred to as the "Madonna"—responded to my request to help the financially struggling clinic, we were thrilled, but we were going to need Ruth's help.

Before committing to anything, Joan was hoping to visit Lee County to get a firsthand sense of the actual conditions and challenges that we and the families faced in East Arkansas. Totally understandable, of course, but the county was hardly a mecca for fine lodging. A few sketchy motels were about the only facilities within a thirty-mile radius of Marianna. That problem was resolved by Ruth Prestridge's kindness and her desire to help the clinic. Without hesitation, Ruth offered up the guest bedroom of her home—an invitation not rescinded when she later found out that Joan would be spending the night with her wildly handsome road manager, Bernie Gelb, *in their guest bedroom*!

Getting Baez to Lee County, Arkansas, was essentially a miracle given her global superstar status at the time, but it was also a lesson for me—that almost anything is possible if you push hard enough.

The idea of convincing Baez to help support our program, a struggling shoestring clinic in this poor and isolated Arkansas county, was the ultimate long shot, but when it became apparent that we were facing existential financial challenges, I needed to do something. Olly was advocating for increased government funding in Little Rock and Washington, DC. We had gone to every foundation and wealthy individual we could get in touch with, and not had much luck.

One Sunday, reading the *Arkansas Gazette*, at that time a very progressive and powerful newspaper, I noticed a short mention of Manny Greenhill, Joan Baez's manager, noting that he was based in Boston. Joan was an A-lister then, of course, with a voice of unparalleled beauty and range. But she was also a serious social activist, pure and almost mythical. It was Joan who discovered Bob Dylan when he was still a very young songwriter and gravel-voiced singer. Joan would bring Dylan, scruffy and raw with his old guitar and beat-up suede jacket, on stage when she was performing and demand that her massive audiences listen to the man destined soon to become legendary himself.

All of this made it highly improbable that I would ever make contact with Joan's manager, no less the superstar herself. But I got Manny's phone number in those halcyon, pre-Google days by simply dialing "information." I called that Monday, and to my enormous surprise, Manny answered the phone. He was gruff and short-tempered, seemingly very bothered—but he took my call.

"Who the hell is this?" Manny barked.

"Thanks for taking the call, sir. My name is Irwin Redlener, and I'm a doctor running a government-sponsored health clinic in a really poor rural Arkansas county, and my clinic is in a bad financial predicament, so . . ."

He interrupted me, saying, "So, why are you calling me?"

"Well, I was hoping to reach Joan and see if she'd be interested in helping us . . ."

"I have no idea," Manny said. "Send me a letter with some information, some details." Click.

That was the conversation. I was too naïve to be intimidated and took the man at his word. I wrote Joan a letter about conditions in the county, about the poverty and the children who were sick and undernourished. I told her that our team of stalwarts and activists needed to stay and make sure people got the medical care they needed. I also put in a couple of eight-by-ten black-and-white photos. One showed a child sitting in a ripped-up easy chair, obviously in a dilapidated shack, and another child, maybe in the same house, sleeping on a rusted bed frame with no mattress or bed coverings. The conditions looked awful, but they were the truth of the whole experience we were living down in Lee County.

I told Karen and Olly about the letter I had sent to Joan Baez. Karen thought that was cool, and I was happy to make a mental note that she really seemed impressed. Olly just kind of grinned. As my "elder" boss and mentor—he was thirty-one, I was a mere twenty-eight at the time—I had trouble reading Olly. He glanced up at the ceiling and shook his head, looking generally amused, I thought. I assumed he didn't think much of my chances of getting a response from Joan, already a global icon. I guess I knew it was pretty much of a long shot, too.

About two weeks later, Baby Sister (I don't think I ever knew her real name), one of the clinic nurses, came into my office and said, "Call for you, Doc. Says her name is Joan and she's calling from California."

I thought, "What the hell? This has to be a joke."

It wasn't.

"Hi, Doc. This is Joan. I got your letter and saw those god-awful pictures. How can I help?"

We talked for ten minutes. I told her who we were and why we were in Lee County. I told her about our financial challenges and how we were desperate for assistance.

She didn't respond right away, and for a minute I thought she had hung up or the call had gotten disconnected.

Then she said, "I will help you, of course. I can do a concert to raise money for the clinic. Probably Memphis would the place to hold the event, but I will discuss logistics with my folks."

I was stunned but totally thrilled. I said, "Joan, that's fantastic. One thing I want to ask. Would you consider visiting us to see for yourself what's going on here?"

Without missing a beat, Joan said, "Absolutely. It's a must."

I couldn't wait to wait to let Olly and Karen know that the incredible, outlandish, improbable thing was going to happen: One of world's most talented and famous artists, the Madonna herself, was going to bail out the Lee County Cooperative Clinic. But not everyone was thrilled that a well-known left-leaning political activist would be paying a visit to our community, a stronghold of white supremacists who already saw the "nigger-loving" VISTA medical team as the advance guard for a communist takeover of the United States.

When word got out that Joan Baez was coming to Marianna, it was clear that she would not be welcomed by many of the white residents of Lee County. These were frustrated and angry people, still and seemingly forever overheated with racism and xenophobia as their cherished traditions were slowly being undermined by forces beyond their control.

So, when I drove Joan and Bernie from the airport in Memphis down State Highway 79, through the run-down hamlets of Greasy Corner and Hughes, through the cotton fields and past the omnipresent shacks, to the outskirts of Marianna, we were greeted with dozens of pickup trucks lining the side of the road. We could see the teeth-gritting faces of angry men, gun racks holding rifles in the back windows of the trucks.

I was astounded by the sight and hoped that this wouldn't rattle Joan. It didn't. She looked out the window, laughing, and said "What the fuck?" while waving sweetly to the stone-faced men who were staring at what they had been told was the she-devil herself, the radical singer who was against everything they stood for. Yes, Joan was a radical and was on the front lines of the protest fight against the Vietnam War. She was a global champion of justice and a civil rights activist who had marched with and sung for the late Martin Luther King, Jr. None of that sat very well with the shotgun-toting welcoming committee of Lee County, Arkansas.

But on that day she was coming to Marianna to help me save the Lee County Cooperative Clinic because its funding was in growing jeopardy, in large part because President Richard Nixon had committed to ending federal funding for VISTA and the community programs supported by the federal government. The LCCC was in the line of fire.

Arkansas has long been a politically enigmatic state. The legendary J. William Fulbright was still a senator from Arkansas when I arrived in Lee County in 1971, and Bill Clinton, the future Democratic president from Hope, Arkansas, was studying at Yale Law School. Fulbright was a segregationist, but otherwise an unrepentant progressive Democrat, renowned multilateralist, enormously respected in policy circles in the United States and abroad—and, of course, namesake of the prestigious Fulbright Scholar Program. Here in the United States, Fulbright's reputation as a free-thinking Democrat was bolstered by his highly vocal criticism of the infamous House Un-American Activities and its right-wing extremist chairman, Joe McCarthy. This was no old-school Southern bigot who clung to segregation as his central theme. Fulbright struggled with his persistent stand on racial separation. Giving him the benefit of the doubt, perhaps he understood all too clearly that to veer from a hard line on segregation would mean no chance of winning an election in Arkansas.

Then there was David Pryor, another liberal Democrat who served in the Arkansas state legislature, the House of Representatives, and the Senate before becoming the state's thirty-ninth governor. Especially noteworthy, finally, was the governor when I arrived in Arkansas, Dale Bumpers. Bumpers went on to run successfully for the U.S. Senate, where he consistently voted with more progressive members of the Democratic Caucus. Besides his congressional duties, Bumpers and his wife Betty built a reputation as staunch advocates fighting for access to health care and immunizations for children, as well as supporting programs critical to the optimal development of young children, especially those living in poverty.

So this was Arkansas. On one hand, there was persistent outright racism, serious poverty, lack of medical care, and terrible, segregated schools in many disadvantaged rural communities. On the other hand, in the second half of the twentieth century, Arkansas repeatedly elected some of the most productive and progressive political leaders to come out of any state.

The Baez visit was simply earthshaking in terms of local reactions and the media. Coverage of her being shown around Lee County by Olly and me was extensive. The concert she had originally proposed actually happened, raising a modest $7,000 or so for the clinic. But that led to something even more productive for our very strained budget. Governor Bumpers, facing severe pressure from white officials in Lee County, had been refusing to release a federal grant that we had been awarded many months prior to Joan's fund-raiser. County government leadership had asserted that we were part of a "communist conspiracy" and should not have access to federal dollars. A letter to the governor from the Lee County dentist, Thomas Cremeen, included these words, referring to my clinic:

This whole thing [the Lee County Cooperative Clinic] is an out an out conspiracy to gain a Communist foothold in a very vulnerable place—and as Mr. Kruschev [sic] himself remarked—perhaps the Communists can take over and never fire a shot.

This was more than a little disconcerting. They were leaning hard on Bumpers, and we were in limbo—until Joan weighed in.

Always the accomplished artist, Joan sketched out a beguiling image of Dale Bumpers leaning over his desk, pen in hand, signing papers releasing our grant, with the caption, "Please sign it!" This was sent by messenger to the governor's mansion in Little Rock. The papers we needed to get the ever-pending grant was signed the next day.

Although the proceeds from the concert were modest, the attention, the extraordinary press, and the active presence of Baez in the Delta gave us access to hundreds of thousands of federal dollars. The clinic would survive an existential threat to its financial stability, even as President Nixon remained committed to dismantling programs like ours across the country.

These experiences did not have the drama and heartbreak of Kent State in 1970, when National Guard troops killed students demonstrating on campus, but saving this vital, remote clinic was a victory in a larger social and political struggle that my generation had taken on. Our work providing health care to the families of Lee County was, of course, always energizing and noble, in a Mother Theresa kind of way. But more important to me was the powerful sense that the team and I were engaged in something much bigger than health care in Arkansas; we were frontline troops in the fight for social justice that was roiling in the early 1970s—exactly where and what I wanted to be.

Working in Arkansas was everything I wanted to do as a doctor. This was where doctors were in terribly short supply, where access to care had been virtually impossible, where medical needs were intense, and where poverty and racism were extreme barriers to meeting basic human needs. This unlikely place is where I felt deeply engaged in issues that mattered. Nothing would be more important to me, back then in Lee County and in the decades that followed.

The House Call

It was a late October afternoon in 1971, just a few months after I arrived in Lee County. The weather was chilly, the sky overcast, the day generally dreary after a couple of days of hard rain, and I was at my desk in the clinic. This is how the day unfolded.

In front of me were stacks of medical charts, a mug half-filled with coffee that was bad enough when it was freshly made several hours ago, probably toxic by this time of the day. I was lost in thought about a child with a heart murmur who had come in a little while ago. He definitely needed to see a specialist, but I was not sure yet how that was going to happen. On the wall behind my desk, thumbtacked onto the cheap paneling, were phone numbers of hospital clinics in Memphis and Little Rock. I had just picked up the receiver of the rotary phone on my desk to start making arrangements for this boy's trip to the big medical center in Little Rock when Anna Mae, one of the nurse's aides, came in to tell me about an emergency call. There was nothing unusual about that; calls came in every day, some serious, others less so. Almost always, though, information from the calls was sketchy at best. Mrs. So-and-so was not feeling too well, "can't hardly get up," or "John tore up his leg in the barn."

This message was different. The caller said a baby was "sick, real sick" and that they lived at a house "pretty far down the road." The nurse who answered the phone did not have a good feeling about this call—and neither did I. It was apparently about a new baby in a house with no phone and, even for Lee County, in a particularly remote location. It was late in the day, and the weather and mud had kept many of the regular patients home, so we were already in the process of closing up for the evening. I decide to head directly over to see this family and check on the sick baby.

It was my first autumn in Arkansas. I had just turned twenty-seven and had been medical director of the clinic for less than three months, still trying to get a feel for unfamiliar terrain— endless stretches of soy and cotton fields, tractors crawling along the two-lane roads, and country folk who would live their lives never venturing more than fifteen or twenty miles from the house where they were born. Interacting with the families about real health issues and making sure they got the best possible medical care was the easy part of this whole experience. Being a doctor was my personal comfort zone, a refuge among Lee County's entirely unfamiliar physical, social, and political realities. The baby we were going to see might be really sick, but I was confident about my skills, what I had been trained to do.

Making a house call was usually pretty straightforward. One of the clinic assistants would drive me to the patient's house, sometimes thirty or forty minutes away from the clinic. On this day, however, the clinic's regular car, a worn-out gray government-issue Ford, was out of commission. George, one of my clinic staff, volunteered to take me in his old pickup truck with a small flatbed and a passenger door that never felt quite securely closed. I grabbed my doctor's bag, and we headed out through Marianna and down Arkansas Highway 79. I tried to make idle conversation with George, but my mind was on that baby; besides, the truck was so noisy we could barely hear each other.

On both sides of the road, even on the main highway west, we passed one decrepit shack after another, almost all with broken porches and tires and rusted auto parts in front. Occasionally, there was an old refrigerator on somebody's rickety porch. The signs of life were shoeless children in tattered clothes near one house, a gray-haired black man waving from the doorway of another shack. We pass a broken-down house trailer, small, dingy yellow, and falling apart, but obviously occupied. Around the side, a very heavy woman was shooing some kids inside, out of the rain, light but steady.

Behind the houses, the soybean and cotton fields looked orderly, newly plowed furrows stretching to the horizon. Huge tractors and harvesters had been left mid-field by the farmers until they returned to work in the morning.

Just before we turned off the highway onto the gravel road, the light rain became a downpour. I glanced at my watch, increasingly anxious to get to this baby. The pickup was doing poorly on the gravel, thrashing and bumping enough to make George as uncomfortable as I was. His grip on the steering wheel was tight, and he was staring straight ahead as we left the gravel road and headed down the last mile on a muddy and narrow lane toward the old sharecropper's shanty at the far end of Lee County, Arkansas.

No more than thirty yards down the dirt road, the truck was in trouble. George was trying to plow through what looked like a small lake just in front of us when the truck came to an abrupt halt. The engine was whining from the strain, but we were not going anywhere, mired in mud almost up to the floorboards and utterly bogged down. "Damn it, George, I've got to get to that patient!" I yelled and, for very unnecessary added emphasis, pounded my fist on the dashboard. Pushing the driver's door open, deep in mud himself, George knew what we had to do. He had his eye on a small farmhouse back on the gravel road where he knew the farmer and would be able to solicit assistance in the form of a tractor and winch.

A half-hour later, we are out of the mud, but I was really worried about the baby waiting for us. For fifteen minutes we slipped and slid, until we got to the house, a miserable, dilapidated shack with a broken-down porch and a door hanging on one hinge. The rain had stopped, but it was now an hour and a half since we set out from the clinic.

I rushed up onto the porch but stepped gingerly on the rotting wood, some of the slats actually missing. I stood for a moment at the doorway, trying to get my bearings. It was dark inside the shack, but my eyes were adjusting enough now to see unpainted makeshift wooden walls. A black potbellied stove was just to the right, and the smell was pungent and musty. Directly in front of me, no more than seven or eight feet away, sitting on a torn, stained mattress on a rusted metal bed frame, the mother held a baby, six or seven weeks old, in her arms. The mother did not take her eyes off the infant, but greeted me very softly. "He's sick." I felt a chill and knew immediately that this baby was, in fact, much sicker than his mother knew. Or maybe she did know, her maternal instincts telling her that this was a terrible situation. I had my bag and walked toward them, saying something in the way of an apology for taking so long to get there. The mother did not respond, but held her sick and very undernourished looking infant up toward me.

This baby was fading; my guess was that he had a bad neonatal infection, but there was no way to prove it in that shack out in the middle of Arkansas nowhere. Back in Denver, where I had just finished my pediatric residency training, this baby would have been transported to a state-of-the-art pediatric intensive care unit. The highly skilled team would have already started an intravenous line, done a lumbar puncture, drawn blood, and hooked up the vital sign monitors.

But this was the backwoods of an impoverished Southern county. My pathetic little doctor's bag held very little that could make a difference here. The walls of this hovel were nothing but rotted wooden boards partially covered with old newspapers to keep out the coming winter drafts. I shook off the feeling of hopelessness to try to do what was possible, in this place, at this moment, for this infant of poverty.

I examined the baby and found what I expected: shallow, rapid respirations and an accelerated heartbeat; skin pale and mottled, with a slightly blueish tinge, as far as I could see in the dimly lit room. The baby felt cool to the touch. I wrapped him for warmth and used a tiny rubber mask and breathing bag to keep him ventilated. We hurried back to the pickup, with me holding the baby and the mother right behind. The ride back to town was interminable, but at least we got through the mud and back onto the highway. In Marianna, we rushed over to the little twenty-five-bed Lee Memorial Hospital, a strange, unfamiliar medical facility that looked and felt like the dusty, impoverished town it tried to serve.

I was no sooner through the emergency room entrance than I was told of two other urgent calls, one from a man not from far from where we had just been. I couldn't believe what was happening. I handed the baby to the nurse and requested immediate transport to Memphis. While we were waiting for an ambulance, I started an intravenous drip on the tiny patient to manage dehydration and start antibiotics. I should have been drawing blood cultures and doing other tests before starting the antibiotics, but the nurse had informed me that there was no infant's lumbar puncture set and they were out of culture bottles. I was enraged, shouting to no one in particular, "What the hell is going on here?"

I last saw the baby being carried onto the local ambulance accompanied by his mother and a nurse from Lee Memorial Hospital. The ambulance sped away, and I stared out toward the highway until it was well out of sight. He would be admitted to an intensive care nursery at the hospital in Memphis—if he made it.

Now where was my driver? I had to get back to the west end of the county; another patient was waiting. At that moment, not far from the Mississippi Delta of East Arkansas and a million miles from anyplace familiar to me, with one year and nine months left of my two-year commitment, I thought: Will I make it?

There was no question that I would make it through my two-year commitment to lead the LCCC. But by April of 1973, Arlene and my sons had been living in Florida for a year, and being so far from David and Jason was increasingly unbearable. As a result, any thoughts I might have been harboring about staying in Lee County beyond June had essentially evaporated. I still needed another year of pediatric training to complete my pediatric specialty requirements; fortuitously, Dr. Bill Cleveland, my old chairman at the University of Miami School of Medicine, offered me a position as chief resident for the academic year 1973–74. (chief resident is a critical role in any clinical department. I would be the official liaison between the residents in training and the departmental faculty and administrators, the chief audiovisual guy, and the person responsible for scheduling all residents through their required rotations.) This situation and opportunity in Miami more or less worked for all of us. I was already supporting Arlene and the boys financially, but now Karen and I would be able to see David and Jason as often as we liked.

Over the last few months, something was definitely happening between Karen and me, to the point that she would be joining me for the move to Florida. Actually, she would be part of my life for everything that would happen from that moment on.

Before leaving Lee County, Karen and I spent a couple of all-night writing sessions producing a proposal to the federal government requesting funds to build a new LCCC facility. The old house in downtown Marianna had served us well as a makeshift clinic for the past three years, but it was much too small to accommodate a rapidly growing clinical practice.

The proposal was successful, and LCCC was awarded $1.2 million dollars. We were gone by the time construction was completed, but Karen and I could not have been happier to leave the clinic with a new facility and an exciting sense of what would be accomplished in the years to come.

Life and Death in the PICU

After my year of serving as chief resident in pediatrics, Dr. Cleveland offered me an opportunity to help design and run the medical school–affiliated Jackson Memorial Hospital's new pediatric intensive care unit, an extraordinary opportunity. I enthusiastically accepted the challenge. It turned into a year of planning and four years of directing a big-city pediatric intensive care unit (PICU), a position about as high pressure as it gets in all of medicine, especially in the mid-1970s when the field was just being recognized as a subspecialty. Ultimately there would be much larger units, not uncommonly twenty to thirty patients in individual rooms receiving various levels of intensive care. Typical staffing in such a large unit would include several attending physicians and teams of doctors in training, ICU specialty nurses, and other support service providers. Importantly, overall responsibility for patient care would be divided among the attending physicians, who also rotated night and weekend coverage.

My unit, brand new in 1974 and filled with the latest technology available, was a relatively large, totally open space with a maximum of eight beds. Every patient admitted to the unit was under my direct care. Few of the other pediatric faculty members were particularly interested in or prepared to take on this responsibility. The singular exception was the pediatric surgeons, for whom the sheer drama and adrenaline rush when a child's life was in the balance were irresistible. I got that. My surgical colleagues, the ICU nurses, an occasional med student, and I spent many all-nighters colluding and collaborating to save the lives of children for whom my unit was the last stop.

The children who came to the ICU were incredibly sick. Some came from our hospital's ER, but many came as transfers from other hospitals in the region where care was all too often horrendous. There were children with intractable asthma, cyanotic and struggling to breathe; children with unrelenting seizures; and those with rare diseases, such as Reye's syndrome, a "new" illness that destroyed the liver and brains of children who had been administered aspirin for high fever associated with certain viral infections. Delays in treatment, wrong medications, and unending cases of outright misdiagnosis were, sadly enough, nearly weekly occurrences.

Dealing with families whose children were extremely ill, their lives literally on the line and needing the most advanced care available, taught me some important lessons about the bonding that can and should occur between the physician and the patients and their families. Under any circumstances, a relationship built on commitment and mutual respect is essential. These are the ingredients of a successful doctor-patient relationship in which children and their families develop trust and confidence in their health care provider. This kind of bonding is an important, highly gratifying aspect of being a physician. It's one of the factors that make caring for people so rewarding and sustaining for many of my professional colleagues.

Typically, in a relationship with a pediatrician, family doctor, or nurse provider, good rapport develops over time. Months or years of interactions lead to trust and confidence that ultimately define the quality of the connection between the doctor and the family. But when a child is critically ill, families are terrified and vulnerable. They need—and sometimes fear—every bit of news about the status of their child. Hardly any experience in life is more unsettling or terrifying than having your child affected by a life-threatening illness or injury. (This our own family knows all too well. In 1999, our then twenty-eight-year-old son Jason died in an accident. We didn't make it to the hospital before he was gone, and we think of him every day—literally a grief that never yields. One of the EMTs who tried to save him reported that his last words were "I'm sorry, Dad." For what, I will never know. But losing a child is an incomparable experience, tempering every other loss one could ever experience—something that no parent should ever have to go through.)

The bonding that occurs between a doctor and a family with a critically ill child happens in an incredibly short time frame. The family must be reassured that their child is in "good hands," being cared for by a team that is not only highly competent medically but compassionate, communicative, and caring. Quality, functional doctor-patient trust in the ICU needs to be established rapidly and authentically, the sooner the better.

There is another aspect of caring for children in intensive care that is not so obvious. In essence, there are ongoing questions regarding whether we, as hard-core, no-nonsense medical staff, should be concerned with the so-called "upstream" causes of life-threatening situations. Why and how did a child end up needing intensive care in the first place? Do we have an obligation—or even the time—to delve into these issues, critical as they might be? A good example of this dilemma was the high prevalence of drowning and near-drowning cases that we saw in our hospital. After all, this was South Florida, where perpetual summer weather and the ubiquitous presence of water was sometimes a deadly mix. There was the proximity of the ocean to the east and south and the warm, inviting waters of the Gulf of Mexico to the west. There were rivers and canals, and perhaps most problematic of all in terms of persistent dangers to children, there were the home swimming pools, so prevalent in all of Florida.

Over and over again we'd see heartbroken and terrified families sobbing with grief or guilt—or both—emerging from the backs of ambulances that had raced through the streets of South Florida bringing in the toddlers who had fallen into the pool, often surrounded by adults enjoying a party, not aware that one of the young children had fallen face down in the water, eventually noticed by one of the guests. Some were resuscitated at the scene, others by the EMTs who eventually arrived. But many never made it to the hospital. Others would be intubated and artificially ventilated, sustaining a heartbeat, but essentially be nonviable because of sustained lack of oxygen to the brain, only to have the "plug pulled" in the ER or in my ICU. Yes, some children would survive the near-drowning and eventually be discharged relatively intact. And we worked like hell to make sure that every child got the best possible opportunity to survive without residual, long-term complications.

But the challenge that went beyond providing critically needed medical care was to what extent we white-coated intensive care medical specialists would, figuratively speaking, venture out of the hospital to deal with the *prevention* of drownings, not just the treatment. Medical care in the hospital—or in any doctor's office, for that matter—is about one-on-one direct health services. Dealing with prevention, the health of populations or communities, and the environmental threats behind the prevalence of any particular medical condition is called "public health."

If it were up to me, every practicing physician would be required to have some training in public health. In the 1970s, doing something about the high prevalence of childhood cases of near-drowning and drowning in South Florida meant seeing ourselves as advocates—public messengers informing parents through the media about water safety, drown-proofing their children, and urging lawmakers to pass regulations requiring pool fencing and other child protection regulations.

And that's precisely what we did. Prevention became our thing. This was from the *Miami Herald* on September 17, 1974. (We had just reported the latest data on drowning and near-drowning cases we had been seeing at Jackson Memorial Hospital):

> "Dr. Redlener says the problem is not one of rescue, but of prevention. . . . 'Laws about swimming pools should be strict and strictly enforced . . . It's like an exposed live wire. You should not be able to leave a swimming pool unprotected.'"

We spoke with parent groups, and we put out material. We reached out to the press and did whatever we could, not just to treat the downstream medical crises but to prevent them in the first place. I was approaching the challenges that confronted my patients in Florida in much the same way as I had in Arkansas, where we were dealing with upstream determinants of health like poverty and contaminated drinking water. We kept a constant eye on the precursor conditions that led to the medical catastrophes that ended up in my ICU. It is this approach, this broad definition of what it means to be a doctor, that has shaped my career ever since.

People like me are "doctor advocates"—aggressive in the ICU, thorough in our patient care, but never reluctant to speak to the public and/or the press. We are purveyors of strong public health messages, exploiting every opportunity to meet health challenges before they emerge as medical emergencies.

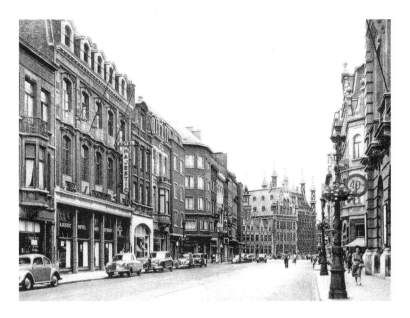

The Majestic Hotel, where I stayed on my first night in Belgium waiting to start medical school, summer 1964. Photo courtesy of the author.

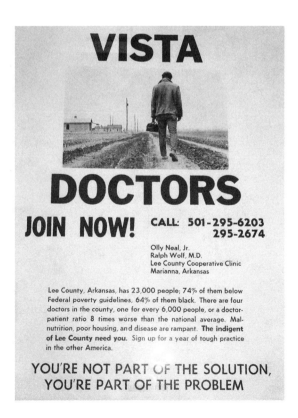

Poster on bulletin board of Denver Children's Hospital that motivated me to drop the pediatric cardiology fellowship and head to the sixth poorest county in America. April 1971. Photo courtesy of the author.

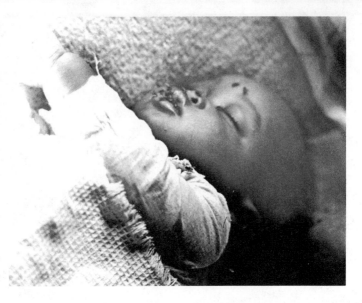

A sick, malnourished infant in Lee County, Arkansas, September 1971. Photo courtesy of the author.

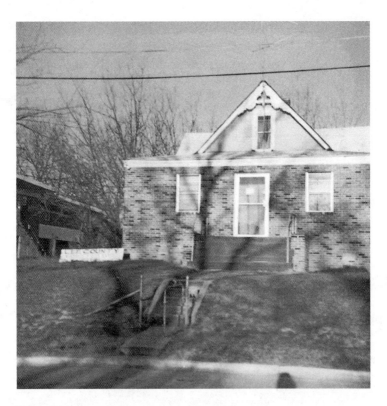

Temporary home of Lee County Cooperative Clinic lent to us by the local undertaker, Lacy Kennedy, until we received federal money to build a new facility. Photo courtesy of the author.

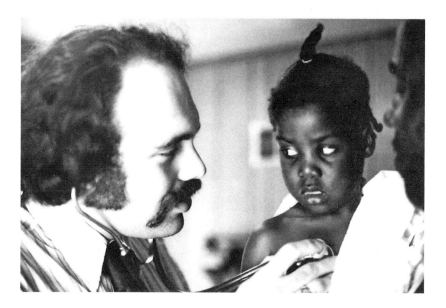

Examining a baby clearly sizing me up, Lee County Cooperative clinic, 1972. Photo by Karen Redlener.

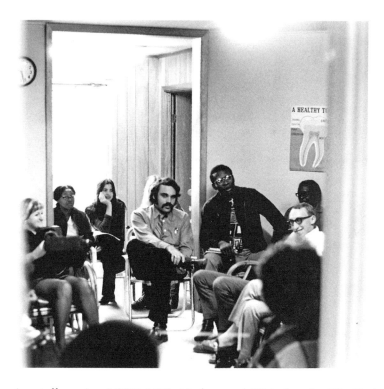

Running staff meeting, LCCC, 1972. My boss and Clinic founder Olly Neal to my left, Karen Redlener to my right. Photo courtesy of the author.

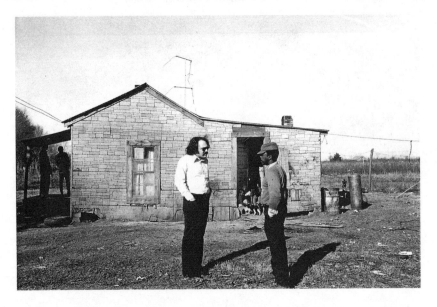

Visiting Walter Patrick's farm, 1972, where I ultimately did my first—and last—operation on a sick hog. Photo by Karen Redlener.

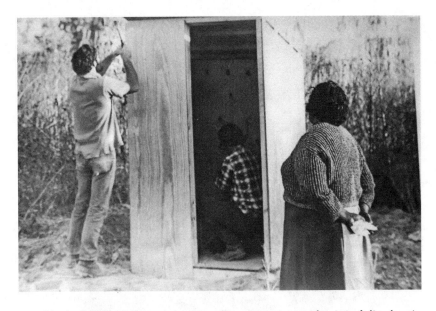

A public health breakthrough in controlling recurring epidemics of diarrhea in Lee County by moving the outdoor privies to a safe distance from the water pumps. Harry Conard, who came up with this definitive idea, was a Vista volunteer with a sanitation engineering background. He's inside the new outhouse being helped by a med student volunteer, overseen by owner of the house, 1973. Photo courtesy of the author.

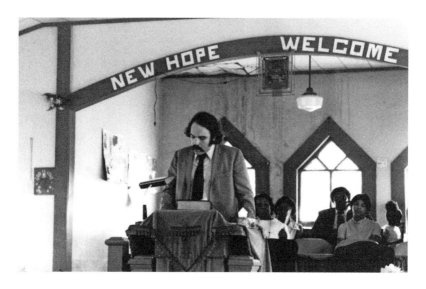

Preaching at a tiny, black Baptist church in Lee County, trying to convince economically disadvantaged citizens that they needed to vote in a new slate of county officials who would be sensitive to their needs. 1973. Photo courtesy of the author.

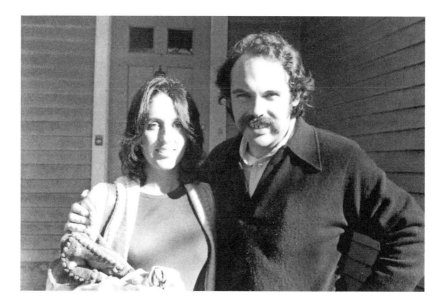

Joan Baez, 1972, visits Lee County preparing to do a benefit concert to keep our program afloat. Photo by Karen Redlener.

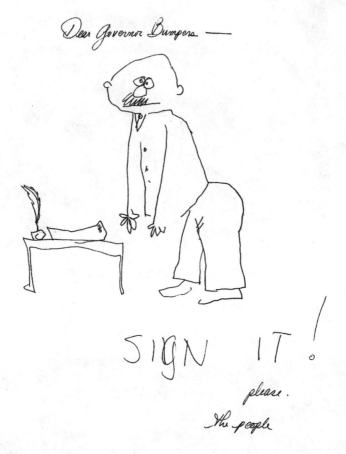

Cartoon sent by Joan Baez to then Governor Dale Bumpers to convince him to sign a federal grant we desperately needed to fund the clinic. He agreed—and we like to think it was due to Joan's very unusual plea.

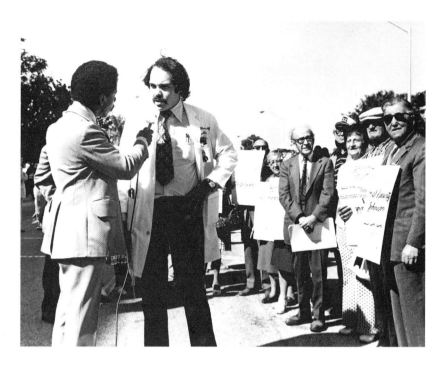

Being interviewed at a health care reform rally in Miami, February 1974. Photo courtesy of the author.

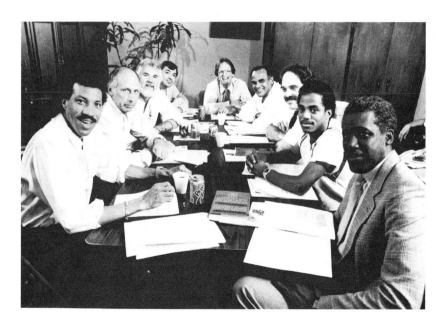

USA for Africa board meeting in 1986. Group shot shows Lionel Richie, Kenny Rogers, Harry Belafonte and Marlon Jackson and others, including L.A. physician soul-mate, Lloyd Grieg. Photo courtesy of the author.

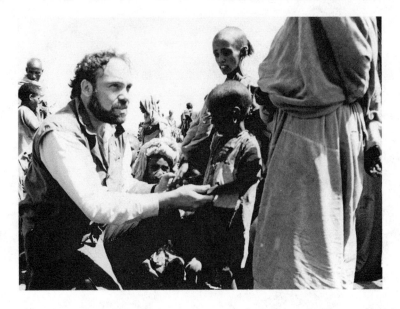

Horrendous scene of illness and starvation in kids during Sub-Saharan drought and famine in 1986. Photo by Dan Farell.

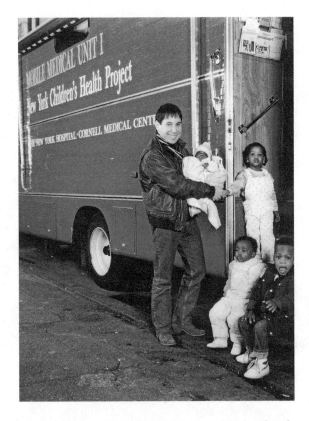

Paul Simon with homeless kids in New York City shortly after first Children's Health Fund project began, late 1987. Photo courtesy of the author.

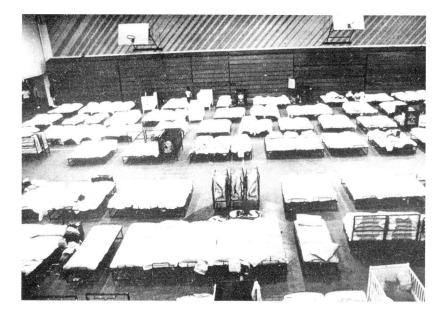

A congregate shelter for homeless families and single adults in the mid-1980s. People would be "sheltered" in such facilities for more than a year under conditions that were horrendously stressful for young children and parents. Photo courtesy of the author.

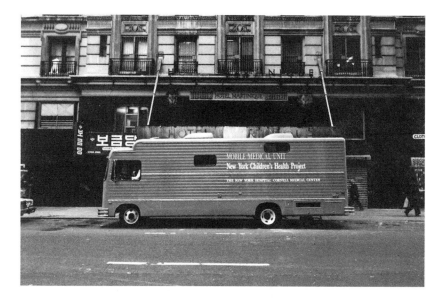

First Children's Health Fund mobile pediatric clinic, custom built after being designed by Karen Redlener, parked in front of the Martinique Hotel in Manhattan. December 1987. Photo courtesy of the author.

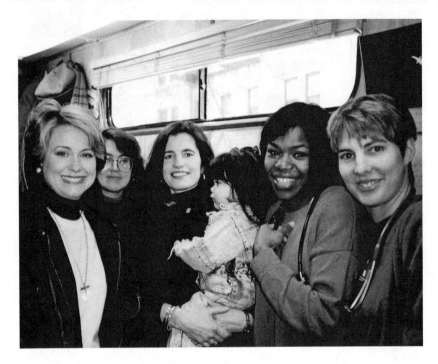

Jane Pauley with Karen Redlener, a young CHF patient, and staffers from New York program, 1989. Photo courtesy of the author.

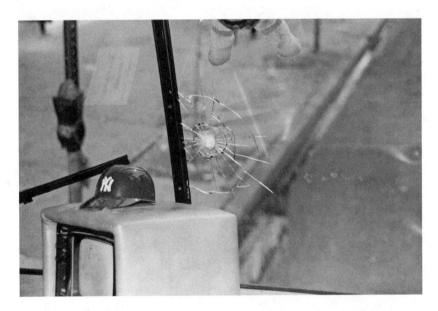

Frightening episode in 1991 when someone fired a 9 mm bullet through the back of the mobile clinic, exiting through the front windshield and narrowly missing a nurse. Paul Simon and I met with the staff, who insisted on serving the same homeless shelter in Brooklyn the very next week. Photo courtesy of the author.

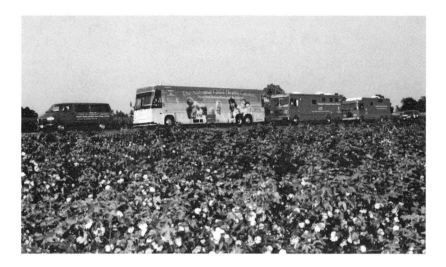

1998. One of two occasions we delivered new mobile clinics to CHF projects in the rural South via caravans stopping along the route for press and speaking events. Photo courtesy of the author.

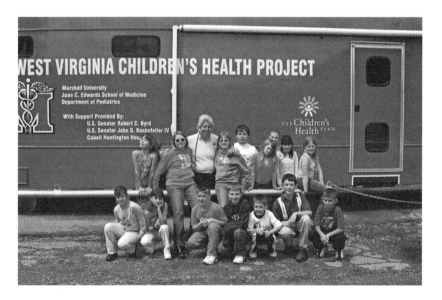

Dr. Isabel Pino, medical director of CHF program in West Virginia, surrounded by a bunch of her patients. Circa 2000. Photo courtesy of the author.

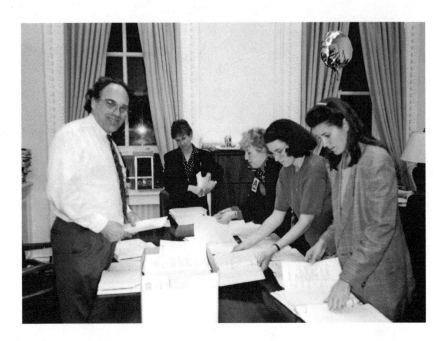

Working with the young, highly talented staff of the Clinton's Health Care Reform Task Force in April of 1993. Photo courtesy of the author.

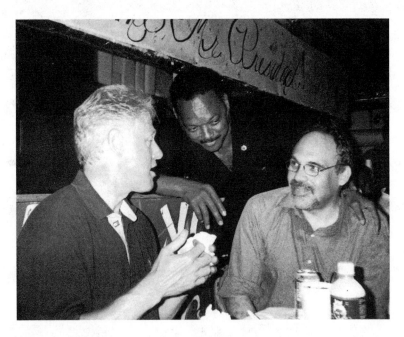

President Bill Clinton, the Reverend Jesse Jackson, and me at a rural Mississippi BBQ joint during the July 1999 national economic development tour organized by the Clinton-Gore Administration. Photo courtesy of the author.

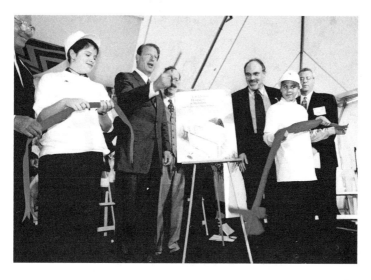

Vice President Al Gore at the groundbreaking for the Children's Hospital at Montefiore Medical Center, South Bronx, 1997. Photo courtesy of the author.

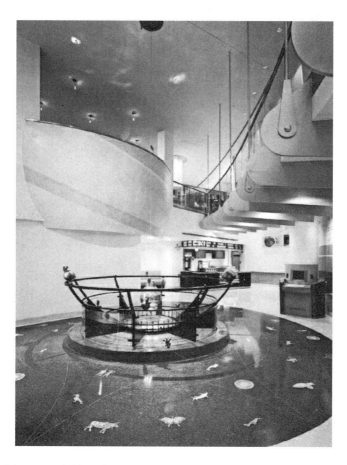

Beautiful interior lobby of the new children's hospital, 2001. Photo courtesy of the author.

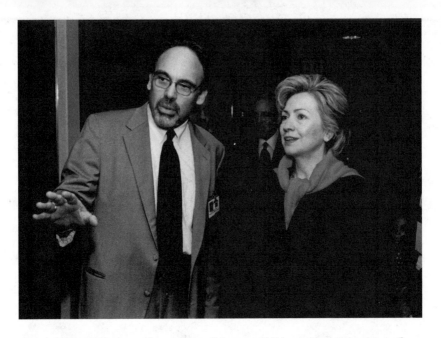

Senator Hillary Clinton at the opening of the new Children's Hospital at Montefiore, 2001. Photo courtesy of the author.

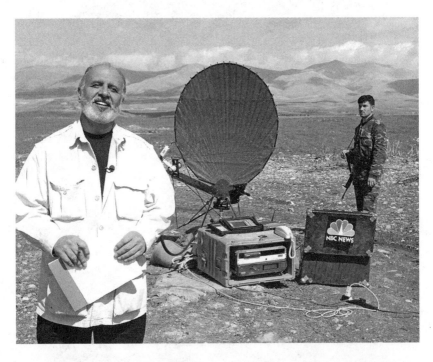

Former NBC senior correspondent and CHF Board member Fred Francis on a live feed to a CHF benefit dinner. Fred was supposed to be in New York making his remarks to our donors but had an urgent assignment in Pakistan. Through modern communications technology, Fred delivered his remarks by satellite in real time. Late 1990s. Photo courtesy of the author.

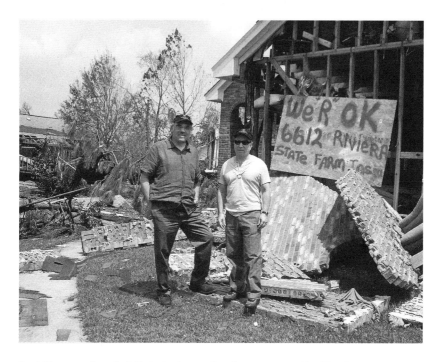

Paul Simon and me in Mississippi assessing damage caused by Hurricane Katrina in 2005. We deployed mobile clinics from CHF's national network. First units and CHF teams were on the ground within days of the storm. Photo by Greg Wilson.

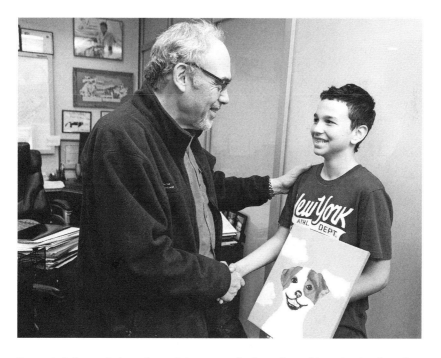

Raymond, formerly homeless adolescent and talented graphic artist, is selected to show one of his paintings at the Metropolitan Museum in New York City. 2014. Photo by Hugh Siegel.

But no matter how much I cared about and pursued advocacy, the constant ebb and flow of patients into the PICU was daunting. Most of the time, I handled the stress with the support of a talented and caring staff. We were able to keep on through the challenges and sadness, doing whatever could be done for every patient, of course, and for the families as well.

Then there was that one child who pushed me to a limit I didn't know I had. It was late December 1977 when a call came into the unit requesting a transfer of a child from a hospital in Broward County, just north of us. The aide at the nurses' station took the call, but a moment later he cupped his hand over the receiver and motioned me over.

"Irwin, I think you better take this call."

He handed me the phone, and the person on the line identified herself as a nurse on the pediatric floor of a community hospital some thirty miles north of Miami. She seemed stressed and anxious, but, as I soon discovered, she had good reason to sound that way. They had a very sick eighteen-month-old boy who "seemed to have circulation problems, and his blood pressure was not stable."

"What do you mean 'circulation problems'?"

"Well, his hands and feet are losing color."

"What are his latest vital signs?"

"Pulse 115, BP 72 over 40, respirations 40."

"Can I speak with his doctor?"

"He's not in the hospital, but he asked me to call and arrange transport to your ICU."

"Well, can I speak with the resident or whoever is caring for him right now."

"No doctor on the floor at the moment."

"I see. Please page the resident or ask the attending to get back to the patient's bedside ASAP. I'll accept the child here, and we'll want to make sure that we get him to Miami in a properly equipped ambulance, accompanied by a doctor and nurse. But first I need to speak to a doctor there who can confirm that the boy is actually stable enough to travel. And I'll need a lot more information about his status and the presumed diagnosis, plus recent lab results and so on."

Three hours later I was standing at the foot of Bed 4 in my ICU. All the other beds were occupied, and I was dimly aware of the cacophony of monitors beeping, staff talking, a couple of babies crying, and an older child calling for her mother. But my focus was on this beautiful blond-haired child being wired up and settled in his bed. He was breathing rapidly but otherwise quiet. Mom was outside the unit, standing in the hallway, having been asked to wait there until we got her son set up. Nurses, aides, and a second-year pediatric resident were working seamlessly, one starting a new IV, another attaching the monitor, still another drawing blood.

I was watching the action, making sure that everything was happening as it should and happening quickly. It was. But something else had me transfixed and anxious. I looked at the toddler's hands. Both were more than "losing color"; his fingers were curled and dark, almost black. I leaned over the foot of the bed, lifted up the white sheet covering his pale legs, and recoiled when I saw the toes of both feet. All of his digits were the same dark ominous color. This boy had gangrene, and this day was going to hell fast.

"Get the surgeon up here, right now," I said to the team. Unless the surgical attending felt otherwise, I was already assuming—correctly as it turns out—that amputations of digits on all four extremities would be necessary, and the procedures would have to be done that day.

This was a tragedy for a one-and-a-half-year-old who would eventually be aware that his physical capacities would be forever limited. What was hitting me especially hard was that the child was of the same age and general appearance as my third son, Michael, now home in South Miami with Karen. I am sure that there were tears in my eyes, and I knew that I wasn't coping well.

And I knew, perhaps more unconsciously than overtly, that my tenure as director of a children's intensive care service needed to be over.

Making matters far worse was eventually getting the whole story of this boy's encounters with the health care system in the week prior to his transfer. There were two visits to his local pediatrician for high fever and diminished "alertness." Both visits were short, the examinations cursory at best, and concluded with reassurances by the pediatrician that he was fine, but "here's a prescription for an antibiotic, just in case."

The third outreach for care was in the ER at the hospital where he was initially admitted. A simple blood test showed very high levels of white blood cells and a pattern consistent with an active bacterial infection. Blood cultures to determine the exact bacteria, which would then guide the specific choice of antibiotic to be given, would have been indicated but were never ordered.

We ultimately got a handle on what had brought this boy to our ICU and led to multiple amputations. He was found to have a very severe blood infection, a disease called meningococcemia, well known to cause cardiovascular shock and gangrene of the extremities if not identified and treated early.

I wish I could say that this was a terrible and unique tragedy. But it was not unique then, and it isn't now. My PICU was in a regional medical center, meaning that very sick children were transferred to us from all over South Florida. I estimated that at least 10 percent of the transferred cases we received had been inadequately treated before being transported to my intensive care unit. Bad medical care was an issue over and over again— and that has not changed very much in the thirty-plus years since. According to a 1999 study by the national Institute of Medicine, "To Err is Human,"[2] nearly 100,000 people die of medical negligence in the United States every year, a particularly heartbreaking situation when the victim is a child.

Poor medical care created an avoidable tragedy for my new patient. That was bad enough, but the fact that this boy was so evocative of my own son pushed a button for me that I would discuss with Karen as soon as I got home—which, as it turned out, was just after sunrise the next day, nearly thirteen hours after the dreaded surgery to amputate his gangrenous digits. Neither the pediatric surgeon nor I left the child's bedside until we were satisfied he was stable enough for us to do so. I asked one of the cardiology attending physicians to cover for me and drove home, wanting badly to share it all with Karen, but I was too exhausted and emotionally drained to do anything but fall quickly asleep on the old sofa we had dragged from our little house in Marianna, Arkansas, an eternity ago.

At Home, in Danger: The Scourge of Abused Children

The transition from Lee County, Arkansas, to Dade County, Florida, had been relatively smooth, though I often missed the rough-and-tumble of caring for a poor community in an environment that felt more like a nineteenth-century segregated Southern community than what one should expect in America in the second half of the twentieth century. That said, any downside of living in South Florida's heat, humidity, and lack of seasonal change was mitigated by the ability to see my boys on a regular basis. That was worth everything.

In many abundantly obvious ways, life and work in Florida could not have more different than living and working in the backwoods of Lee County. Miami, a bustling, bilingual, bicultural metropolis had the culture, the buzz, and the glamour of a rising urban force; rural Arkansas was an impoverished, forgotten corner of a region that could easily be seen as on the very brink of absolute hopelessness.

Yet I was struck by some commonalities between the urban vibrancy of Miami and the rural isolation of Lee County. Hard-core rural poverty with shacks, outdoor privies, swarming flies, and barefoot babies on the front porch were the images from my time in Arkansas. Miami's inner-city neighborhoods were the urban version of severely disadvantaged communities: city blocks rife with crime, drugs, and sullen despair. Both places had their share of deep-seated poverty—one seen in abandoned plantations and soybean fields, the other in downtrodden homes and run-down schools. In essence, poverty is poverty, in terms of the impact on children and families. Both environments had inordinate numbers of children who were marginalized because of race and/or economic disparity.

As far as I could see, neither Dade County nor Lee County showed any real interest in understanding or addressing the needs and aspirations of children who were struggling. Both communities, as different as they could be, were doing a very poor job of protecting children who were acutely suffering. In Arkansas, people would bring undernourished infants to my office in infant carriers made of cardboard boxes; in Miami, battered and abused kids were brought in by ambulance to my hospital's emergency rooms and the pediatric intensive care unit. In both places, too many children were starting off life already behind, with too many impediments to surviving childhood with their dreams and potential intact.

Among the issues I took on as a junior faculty member in Miami was the challenge of preventing and treating child abuse and neglect, a professionally complex and emotionally charged issue that many of my colleagues avoided at all costs. This was an issue that I found highly compelling, in no small part due to the influence of Dr. Henry Kempe in Denver, who had been such an inspiration during my training.

In the early 1970s, child maltreatment was neither sufficiently recognized nor reckoned with by government officials or the public in general. The media would cover a dramatic case of gross abuse, as it would any horrific crime story, but not as the social and public health challenge that it actually was. As a result, little was happening in the way of programs or resources to prevent child abuse or treat the families who were caught in the cycle of poor parenting skills, isolation, and domestic violence. We needed a breakthrough—some way of getting the public and policy makers to focus on this horrendous issue and begin taking on the challenge of breaking the cycle of abuse and neglect that was affecting the lives and futures of at least a million children every year in the United States. We had to find a way to put this whole issue on the front burner for policy makers—and the public.

The answer involved "going public" with a very clear message about the nature of child abuse and neglect, and what needed to be done. To help think this through, I turned to a close friend and one of the most effective broadcast journalists in the region, WCBS correspondent Fred Francis. Fred was intrigued by the issue and immediately grasped the notion of a real wake-up call for the public and policy makers. We both understood that child abuse was a seriously underappreciated social and public health problem. We needed a plan and came up with one in short order.

The plan, in essence, was that I would track emergency room intake at Jackson Memorial Hospital and call Fred immediately after contacting social services when the next serious abuse case showed up. If Fred and his crew could get there before the social service workers, he could start filming and interviewing before being he told he was not allowed to see, no less photograph, an abused child. Our plan was to convince the officials that getting this story out would be a major public service—ultimately saving lives.

One humid night in June 1974, James showed up in the Jackson Memorial pediatric ER. The three-year-old was wide-eyed and terrified, with multiple bruises and burns everywhere on his body. Even seasoned medical staff were stunned and distressed seeing the visible evidence of what this little boy had endured. James's aunt had brought him to the hospital. His mother had accompanied them, but she was too distraught to be questioned and had been immediately sent to the crisis intervention unit just outside the ER. The staff called social services—and I called Fred. As planned, the fearless journalist was there in moments and had already begun filming before the social workers got to the scene.

I was well aware of the ethical dilemma I was creating. Long before explicit regulations were in place, I was very concerned that we would be filming a child without formal permission. On the other hand, child abuse was an unrecognized epidemic. Nobody was paying attention. If we were going to make changes and try to stop rampant abuse and neglect, we had to make the general public and elected officials sufficiently aware of what was going on to demand action. Amazingly, the social service team didn't really protest the TV coverage. I believed they were as concerned as we were that child maltreatment was so rampant, with very little evidence that public officials were addressing—or even recognizing—this crisis.

So Fred just continued reporting. For five evenings, the Miami CBS affiliate news anchor spoke soberly, preparing viewers for what they were about to see. Each evening, he recommended that viewers send "children and other sensitive persons" out of the room while the segments aired—and for good reason. This would be one of the most riveting and horrifying broadcasts Miami viewers had ever seen. With relentless focus and graphic footage, it took on the issue that society had been avoiding: how and why so many children were being abused and what we would have to do to stop this raging epidemic.

The first segment opened with Fred reporting live from my pediatric ICU—the first telecast of this kind in South Florida. He stood by James's crib, and the camera began to focus in on the young boy, swaddled in white bandages.

"In Dade County," he began, "we are killing, neglecting, and abusing our children at a chilling rate. Now, we know this better than most of our nation, not because our citizens are sicker or more barbaric, but because we keep excellent records."

"Yet," added, "that is all we do."

As the camera zeroed in during my examination, I gently turned James around and pointed out crescent-shaped bruises, several days old, most prominently on his left shoulder but also elsewhere, likely caused by blunt trauma—maybe a belt. I pointed to other injuries that appeared to be more recent, including some unexplained facial bruises.

I carefully placed him on the floor, kneeling down to continue the exam.

"James, can you get this?" I asked, placing his bottle a few paces away. I wanted to see him walk. I had learned this from Henry Kempe, chairman of pediatrics and my mentor during training in Denver. The point was that a child's gait would often reveal problems that were not otherwise visible, including broken bones or dislocations. There was nothing of concern there, but when the nurse and I tried to remove James's diaper, he whimpered in protest—and with good reason.

Between his buttocks was an ugly red, blistering burn. Fred's camera was still running. I noted that the injury did not look like the typical immersion burn from being deliberately placed in scalding water—an all too common form of painful abuse. If it had been immersion, the burns would have covered the buttocks and genitals—and that was not the case here.

As the camera focused in on the blistered, raw lesion, I told Fred and everyone watching this exam unfold that the burn was likely caused by a hot object thrust between his buttocks. Something like a hot curling iron could have caused what we were seeing.

I turned James around and discovered another shocking image: evidence of sexual or genital abuse, with scratches and scarring of the toddler's penis.

James knew who had done this to him.

"James, honey, who hurt you?" I asked the boy after placing him back on an examining table. At first, the nurse and I couldn't understand his response, but he continued straining to express himself.

"Mommy," he was saying. "Mommy hurt."

As photos of horribly abused children from Jackson Hospital flashed on the screen, Fred cited the shocking statistics—in the past twelve months, six children had died as the result of child abuse, twenty-six had had their skulls fractured, forty-three children had suffered broken bones, sixty-one had been starved, and sixty-eight had suffered terrible burns from cigarettes, scalding liquids, and hot stoves.

It was gruesome, a one-two punch of James's story and a rundown of the national statistics. In fact, it's worth noting that in 2016 a news organization would not be permitted to broadcast these graphic videos involving a child—perhaps rightly so. But the publicity from a case decades ago had the desired effect. The public was generally horrified by the images, and public officials accelerated plans to find new ways of identifying and preventing the abuse of children.

One of the most salient outcomes of the press coverage for me was a spontaneous call from Steve Green, a young Miami-based businessman and philanthropist who wanted to know what he could do: "I want to help you—what do you need?"

"I need the resources to start a program to save children and help families break the cycle of abuse."

"Done," he said.

Six months later we started the Child Action Project, the region's first program of its kind. The program gave us the resources to train professionals to better identify potential abuse and neglect cases and to establish an office and staff dedicated to the program. But the constant flood of abused and neglected children coming to our hospital continued.

In 1976 a fourteen-month-old girl was admitted to the pediatric intensive care unit with multiple bone fractures and evidence of bruising around the buttocks as well as on her arms and legs. She was not "in extremis" but clearly had been severely physically abused over a period of many months prior to her admission. The rest of the history, as far we could obtain it, was fairly unremarkable, but what got my attention was the child's first name: Precious.

Apparently her parents, Pamela and Johnny, really did consider the child "a gift," at least when she was first born, so they chose a name they thought was sweet and descriptive. However, neither mother nor father had any real sense of normal child development, behavior management, or the most basic information necessary to appropriately raise a child. Both parents were themselves raised in dysfunctional homes; Johnny's was physically abusive, Pamela's detached and neglectful.

The question was, where did they learn about parenting at all? After extensive interviews with the parents, it became clear that what little information they did have about raising a child was highly uninformed, picked up from social connections who knew even less than they did. Trouble began in earnest as Precious started "disappointing" her parents.

"Precious didn't stop crying no matter what we did or said!"

First they tried feeding her more often and even "talking her down," as they said. but that didn't work to control what was likely a case of infant colic.

Pamela said, "Johnny would come home from work, yelling at *me* for not controlling the baby. He was under tremendous stress from a lousy job and a terrible boss." All of that drama caused increasing stress for Pamela, and, as the tension rose, so did her anxiety. She was desperate to do "whatever it would take to get that baby to quiet."

According to a woman she met in a local bodega when Precious was five months old, a baby like that could be "taught." A little spank would help the baby "learn" that she had to control herself. Having no relatives or close friends she could rely on to get other perspectives, Pamela did what the stranger in the deli suggested. First it was smacks on the diapered backside, which, needless to say, did little to stop the colic attacks.

"Did you ever discuss what to do with your baby's doctor?" I asked.

"What doctor? We had no money for regular doctors, and Johnny and me couldn't qualify for welfare," Pamela responded.

"So, where did she go when she needed medical attention?" I asked.

"Whatever emergency room was closest," Johnny said. "Usually, down in South Miami, but we tried not to go to the same place too often, since we couldn't afford to pay the bills."

Before long the backside spanks turned into harder slaps on the baby's legs, eventually much harder smacks to the chest and occasionally her face. The bruises were becoming noticeable. As the baby grew older, more issues were emerging. Right around Precious's first birthday, Johnny came home upset and frustrated. Somebody at work had bragged about his baby learning to walk at age eleven months. The truth is that most babies do take their first steps between nine and twelve months, and many are fairly proficient walkers by twelve to fifteen months. That said, many perfectly normal babies delay walking until sixteen months or so.

But to Johnny and Pamela, this developmental delay was another provocation by a baby who didn't seem to "get it." The parents concluded that what Precious needed was "walking training"— a brainstorm concocted on their very own. One of them would hold the baby's hands while the other, on the floor, moved the child's feet.

"Walk, Precious. Walk, God damn it!" Johnny would say— clearly with no effect. That frustration led to more and more severe physical abuse. The infant's bones showed fractures; some seemed "fresh" when she was finally admitted. Other healing fractures of varying ages were evident.

When Precious showed up at the pediatric emergency room lethargic, whimpering, and covered with bruises, the staff in my teaching hospital knew exactly what they were dealing with; they ordered full body x-rays and basic blood work and asked for a direct admission to the intensive care unit. And that's where I came to meet this terribly abused child and her sad, bewildered, and very dysfunctional parents, who had neither the insights nor the skills nor any ability to know how to facilitate a baby's successful trajectory through a positive childhood.

Precious's physical injuries eventually healed, but what became of her emotionally I never learned.

Fast-forward to late June 2016. I was in a fashionable Upper West Side Manhattan grocery store, picking up some blueberries and milk. Just in front of me in line was a well-dressed thirty-something mother with three children in tow. The two older girls, who looked to be perhaps about five and seven years of age, were giggly and very focused on each other. Then there was the rambunctious little boy, probably four years old. He was a bit out of control—hardly a felony for a child his age—but the mother was beside herself.

I was watching and listening intently; she was smiling, a kind of teeth-gritting fake smile, and calling her son.

"Andrew. Get over here! Damn it, Andrew, what's wrong with you?"

Andrew was unprepared to answer that question, so he continued running up and down the frozen foods aisle. He opened the ice cream freezer and yelled out to his mother, "I want ice cream! You said I could have ice cream."

"Not you," his mother responded, clearly furious. "Your sisters are getting ice cream. They're good. You are a very bad boy. You always are, and you may never get ice cream again if you don't start behaving," she threatened him.

Now he ran over to her, essentially wailing. I was feeling her palpable frustration—or was it just embarrassment, as all eyes in the store were now on the drama by the checkout counter? As soon as little Andrew got close enough to grab, the mother got his right upper arm in a vice grip and was almost frothing as she continued to verbally berate the boy.

"Mommy, stop! You're hurting me. Stop, Mommy!"

Now I was getting concerned. Pediatricians (along with teachers, social workers, and certain other child care professionals) are actually "mandated reporters." If we see a child obviously being abused—in any material way—we are required to "call it in." I found myself struggling to remember whether that legal obligation only applied to children that I was seeing professionally. What about an encounter like this in this upscale store in an affluent New York neighborhood? Did the legal mandate mean "any child in trouble, anywhere"?

Meanwhile, Andrew squirmed from his mother's grip. She managed to grab onto his shirt, nearly lifting him off the ground.

"Mommy, you're tearing my shirt. I'm scared."

"Think you're scared now? How about I send you back to Aunt Debbie?"

"No. No, I don't want to go there again. She's mean, Mommy."

The mother called out to her older daughters. "Take this monster outside," she commanded them. Her face was flushed, and she was doing everything possible to avoid eye contact with the increasingly interested and, I imagined, concerned audience of fellow shoppers. Meanwhile, I had slipped over to an adjacent checkout lane and was able to pay and leave the store just before Andrew's mother left through the main exit. Once outside, I made a decision not to call "the agency," but I was anxious to speak with this mother.

"Hi. I know you probably think this is entirely none of my business, but I am a pediatrician and a grandfather, so I want to give you some heartfelt, though I know unsolicited, advice." I was

143

talking fast, not having any idea how long it would be before this stranger would punch me in the face or just walk away.

She smiled weirdly, perhaps a bit curious, who knows? Whatever she was thinking, she stopped and at least looked interested, so I launched right in.

"Listen, you clearly have a very active little boy who must be a real challenge to manage. But what I often tell parents of kids like this are three things:

"First, I don't know you or your kids, but I will tell you that many entirely normal three- or four-year-old boys can indeed be very active; they are not necessarily "hyperactive" in a diagnostic sense, and certainly not 'bad.'

"Second, you must choose your battles. If you treat every behavior he exhibits as equally out of control or evidence of serious disobedience, there is no way he'll be able to distinguish among the things you're trying to correct. If minor infractions get the same anger reactions from his mom as do more serious behaviors, it's all an emotional blur, and that just neutralizes what you're trying to accomplish.

"Third, try this: Lovingly praise Andrew when he does something that's reasonably—and relatively—something you'd call good behavior. If you give him negative feedback when he gallivants down the aisle, praise him lavishly if he's standing next to you, relatively calm, even if he's fidgety. That can help a lot."

I would like to think that she listened and learned, but I really have no idea if my words had any effect at all. At least I didn't get slugged—and she didn't storm away.

Utica to Addis Ababa: Face to Face with a Major Catastrophe

After five years of pediatric intensive care, public health projects, training physicians, teaching students, and academic research,

I badly needed a break. What lay in store going forward was not entirely clear, but Karen and I were up for something very different. To the surprise of virtually everyone who knew us, we headed north to Utica, New York, where I first joined a group practice as one of four pediatricians and later opened my own practice in an office building attached to one of the major regional hospitals in upstate New York.

Karen helped set up the practice and managed all of its administrative tasks. Meanwhile, the family was growing fast. By 1980 we had two young children, Michael and Stephanie. Two years later my older sons, fourteen-year-old David and twelve-year-old Jason, moved up from Florida, and suddenly we were raising four children. Fortunately, the community could not have been more welcoming, helping us orient, make the right connections, and generally adapt to life upstate. For the kids, Karen, and me, some of our still closest friends are those we met there in Utica, an economically struggling community in the foothills of the Adirondacks that welcomed us with open hearts.

The practice was a booming success. As the only pediatrician in the community with intensive care experience, I was given the responsibility of overseeing the hospital's newborn ICU. It was nothing like the experience I'd had in Miami in terms of size or scope; babies who required ongoing intensive care would be transferred to a larger academic center, mostly to the teaching hospital in Syracuse. Still, for the first few years, practicing in Utica was busy and rewarding—and exhausting. I was called on and available at all hours, seven days a week, when a baby was in serious medical trouble.

My practice was increasingly populated by children with complex or serious chronic illnesses—challenges of diagnosis and management that I found stimulating and rewarding. Tough case? Bring it on! Maybe I was/am an adrenaline junkie with a stethoscope. And maybe I didn't mind the fact that I became a local "medical celebrity" of sorts, well known in the community, the go-to doc for the most difficult and urgent pediatric emergencies.

Then, too, while I was in an exceedingly busy community practice, there was never a time when I wasn't involved in activism and advocacy around issues beyond the care of my patients, a responsibility I took very seriously. Connecting with kids, bonding with families, and managing complex medical challenges energized my interest in the practice. But beyond clinical care, I continued to be drawn to other work, including collaborating with colleagues at the medical center in Syracuse on organizing a referral system for sick and premature infants.

My biggest external involvement was chairing the national executive committee of Physicians for Social Responsibility (PSR). In the late 1970s and through most of the 1980s, PSR was focused on one thing: informing the public and policy makers about the existential danger posed by the ever-expanding arsenal of powerful nuclear weapons being accumulated by the world's superpowers, primarily the United States and the Soviet Union.

The iconic American public health pioneer, Dr. Jack Geiger, a principal founder of PSR, was one of the physicians who inspired so many of us to get involved in high-energy public health advocacy. Jack was a major role model for wannabe doctor advocates, including me. In fact, Jack was surely my most influential mentor, and eventually he and his double-PhD wife, Nicole Schupf, became dear friends of mine and Karen's. Besides his powerful voice in the anti-nuke movement, Jack had pioneered the idea of community health centers for indigent urban and rural populations. We modeled our own program in Lee County, Arkansas, in part on the groundbreaking work Jack did to establish the nation's first rural community health center in Mound Bayou, Mississippi. It was there that Jack famously wrote prescriptions for food when his impoverished patients faced nutritional deficiencies and persistent hunger. Jack believed that treating hunger and dealing with grinding poverty were as important for physicians as was prescribing antibiotics for strep throat.

In our roles with PSR, Jack and I were among a cadre of physicians who traveled the world, testified before Congress, and pressed the media to cover our unified statement of concern—that if nuclear war broke out, the consequences would threaten all life on the planet. Human fatalities and injuries would be overwhelming to the point where no medical response could be possible, so our only recourse was to prevent nuclear war in the first place. That meant dealing with policy makers, elected officials, the media, and collaborators in every nuclear nation in the world.

In Utica I was regularly outspoken about issues that were far outside the bounds of children's health; the nuclear arms race was a good example. This was unusual, to say the least, for a physician in upstate New York. I was getting substantial local media coverage, to the point where the Democrats asked me to consider running for Congress in 1984. I actually considered—albeit briefly—running for the then-vacant seat representing New York's Twenty-Second Congressional District. Karen said absolutely no way, leaving no room for discussion. Yes, I was intrigued, but Karen knew that I would be deeply frustrated for many reasons, not least of which was the nonstop fund-raising and campaigning for reelection every two years.

The fact that I even considered such an option was calling the big question: where exactly was I headed? Was I a practicing doctor or a public health activist and advocate? Yes, I was enjoying my practice, and I certainly wasn't bored. To the contrary, I was happy to set up a practice and enjoy a meaningful, almost quaintly normal, family life there with Karen and our kids. But I was getting restless, missing working with disadvantaged children and working on large-scale public health challenges. Every year it was getting increasingly difficult to imagine a lifetime commitment to community-based private practice so far from the "action" (wherever and whatever that might be).

The idea of getting out of that town and on to the next thing really crystalized one early morning as I was making "baby rounds" at St. Luke's Hospital. In a typical scenario for a pediatrician, I was sitting at the nurses' station writing notes on the newborns I had just examined. I looked up from the chart and saw an older man, draped in a sterile gown, hunched over a bassinet checking out one of the babies. The doctor was one of my colleagues and a friend, Dr. Arthur Kaplan, at that point eighty-one years old—almost forty years older than I was. Kaplan was a smart doctor, great with patients and very involved in political advocacy. He had helped me form the local chapter of Physicians for Social Responsibility.

But I wasn't only seeing the venerable Arthur Kaplan, revered dean of the pediatric community in Utica. What I saw was my own future: Dr. Redlener, forty years hence, leaning over a baby in the newborn nursery for the 10,000th time, chatting with the new mothers, reiterating routine feeding advice, telling the same old jokes, trying to be charming, and wanting to sound experienced and competent. The whole picture terrified me. I felt as though I was staring into a future that I wanted no part of. I couldn't let that happen.

That was a revelation that I couldn't wait to share with Karen. She smiled when I told her that we had to get out of Utica. As much as she saw Utica as a good place to raise our children, she was also looking for new challenges, particularly fulfilling her long-held aspiration of getting a masters degree. She clearly understood what I was saying, later telling me that she was confident I would figure out a meaningful transition for me and the family. In fact, that transition was about to begin, strangely enough, because of a terrible public health calamity unfolding in sub-Saharan Africa, some 7,000 miles from my office at St. Luke's Hospital in Utica, New York.

In 1984 the drought and resulting famine that affected Ethiopia, Sudan, and most of their neighboring countries was epic by any standard. Ultimately at least one million men, women, and children would die of starvation and disease. The world was about to understand what was at stake and that the response needed to be massive, global, and sustained. In December 1984, deeply troubled by what he had seen in Africa, British rock star Bob Geldorf produced a heart-wrenching hit song called "Do They Know It's Christmas?" and a double-venue concert involving some of the UK's most prominent pop singers, with all proceeds going to hunger relief efforts.

Within a few months of Live Aid, the legendary singer-activist Harry Belafonte helped create the U.S. equivalent of this effort by setting up an organization called USA for Africa (USAFA). Belafonte had been involved with African political and social issues since the late 1950s. He was a major figure in the antiapartheid movement and one of the early leaders of the Peace Corps, working hard for this agency in both Africa and Washington, DC. Harry was recognized as the main driver of USAFA, one of the most successful celebrity-driven charitable efforts of all time.

In early 1985, Harry asked Michael Jackson and Lionel Richie to write USAFA's theme song, which they titled "We Are the World." Quincy Jones produced and recorded the record at a secret location in Hollywood, where he gathered more than forty of the most famous pop stars in the world, including Paul Simon, Bob Dylan, Diana Ross, Ray Charles, Bruce Springsteen, Tina Turner, and many more. Regular play on almost every radio station in the United States led to enormous sales, and the record eventually earned some $60 million that would be directed to famine relief in sub-Saharan Africa.

Like so many people around the world, I was riveted by the ongoing tragedy and saddened to see the faces of starving children. Other than buying the record, I was committed to figuring out what more I could do.

Then, in March of 1985, once again a serendipitous opportunity presented itself in an examining room of my pediatric office.

149

It was billed as a routine appointment with a new patient. A young boy and his mother were there for a "get to know you" visit, the family having just moved from New Jersey. By sheer coincidence, "We Are the World" had been released the week before I met this new family and was already a megahit. The media focus, not just on the song but on the crisis in Africa, was such that, for whatever reason, the mother and I talked about it during our social chit-chat. Then she dropped a casual comment that immediately got my attention.

"You know, I have a brother I am very proud of. He's actually a very talented musician who happened to have played percussion for the "We Are the World" record, the mother said.

"Really?" I said "You mean he was actually in that secret location where every major pop star showed up?"

"Exactly."

Now it was off to the races. The mother put me in touch with her brother in Los Angeles, and he in turn connected me to Marty Rogol, USAFA's executive director. Some two weeks later, I was meeting with Marty in New York City, discussing USAFA's plans, and offering to help in any way I could.

"We are, for sure, raising a lot of money," Marty said, "and we hope to do a lot of good for people being affected by this terrible crisis. It is really important that we do this right. We want to spend the money quickly and responsibly, with real accountability."

"Yes, of course," I said.

"Plus, the artists themselves who produced and performed on 'We Are the World' have a lot on the line. This has to be a charitable project that actually understands what's at stake, helps people, and, at the end of the day, is something that the artists can be proud of."

"Understood. So how can I help?"

"Well, right now we have a lot of enthusiasm and a terrific organization under development, but we don't enough have people on board who understand the actual health and nutritional needs of the famine victims, especially the children. And we don't have the technical expertise to properly evaluate the hundreds of requests for funding we are already receiving from organizations working in the field. Do you think you can help with any of this?"

I looked at Marty, trying to evaluate exactly what I might bring to the table. While in Miami, I had helped lead a large-scale medical response to a major natural disaster, the Guatemalan earthquake in 1976. I had also organized and led several trips to Honduras with medical students to teach them about health and nutrition in low-resource environments. Most important, while it was not an international setting, my intense two years of working in Lee County, Arkansas, were pretty close to a Third World experience.

"Sure. I would be honored to help any way I can," I said, even though I had no idea how I would manage this in an already very busy life, with my nonstop pediatric practice in Utica, my work and travel schedule with PSR, and, of course, Karen and the four kids. But we had already been processing the fact that we were psychologically ready to leave Utica and the practice, and I had enough self-awareness to understand that my life, my work, and the shaping of my personal mission were being driven by an exquisite sensitivity to the excitement, the pure adrenaline rush, of embracing serendipity. This opportunity that Marty Rogol had just laid out was clearly one of those unexpected moments—which is why my processing of Marty's request took about two seconds.

"Of course," I responded, "I'd be honored to help make this all happen."

Three months later, I found myself on a high-visibility trip organized to deliver a jumbo jet full of relief supplies to a ring of African countries overwhelmed by famine and disease. The plane left from Los Angeles, picked me up at JFK airport in New York, and flew to Brussels, where it was loaded with supplies that included a ton of high-nutrition biscuits. Michael Jackson's brother Marlon was already with us, along with a couple of other USAFA leaders, including Los Angeles physician Lloyd Greig; Belafonte would be joining us at the stopover in Brussels.

Lloyd, a well-known and beloved Hollywood-based obstetrician, brought great energy and expertise to the team. Lloyd and I bonded quickly as we traveled together on the initial trip delivering supplies to Ethiopia and Sudan. We shared witness and commiserated, sometimes stunned and horrified, other times laughing and processing what we were seeing in ways that only fellow doctors can do—meaning not always appropriate and generally not easy for nondoctors to appreciate.

Every day of the trip, we were up early visiting ministries, attending relief worker debriefings, or visiting barely functioning hospitals and remote villages. Even in Addis Ababa, Ethiopia's capital, home to the country's most prominent teaching hospital—the Black Lion—we saw wards full of children with malnutrition and the full gamut of diseases endemic in poor countries, including rheumatic fever, rickets, stunted growth, and lethal cases of the measles. In the primitive neonatal intensive care nursery, we watched as the hospital staff switched the single oxygen tank among a dozen babies struggling to breathe, many of them too premature or too overwhelmed with infection to survive.

In the rural communities of Ethiopia and Sudan, we walked through the sweltering corridors of facilities barely meriting the label "hospital"—strings of huts or small adobe buildings containing mostly dark and dirt-floored patient rooms where worried relatives did the best they could to provide basic nursing care, food, and needed medications for their sickly, forlorn children.

What we saw everywhere was suffering and profound sadness, overwhelming the senses and bringing some of us to tears. The visit to a refugee center in Mekele, in northern Ethiopia, was paralyzing in scale. Seeing, holding, interacting with sick and starving children was irresistible for most of us. Makeshift lean-tos sheltering bedraggled and hungry migrants coming down from the drought-stricken hills were interspersed with field hospitals stood up in tents to care for dying patients—all of it underscoring the insufficiency of the response to this remarkable humanitarian crisis.

While we were in-country we learned of a massive delivery of brand new 12-foot diameter tents donated by a group of Europeans. This was seemingly a great gift and a welcome opportunity to improve the conditions for the hundreds of thousands of displaced families gathering in Mekele. But not long after the delivery and deployment of the tents, relief organizations began noticing that the mortality rate among malnourished children was rising fast.

What was going on? Infection and contagion rates seemed stable. This medical mystery was eventually solved when an astute public health professional figured out that the problem had to do with delay in identifying the sickest children who needed urgent care, including hydration. Prior to the tents being set up most families sheltered under a few cloth or burlap sheets held up by a single pole. So when relief workers walked through the camp they could easily see children who were in bad shape and get them to one of the hydration units. But when the tents were in place, children were out of sight. By the time it was realized that a child was in critical condition, it was often too late to save him.

Every challenge we faced was complicated by brutal politics. Mengistu Haile Mariam was the military and political leader of Ethiopia during the great famine. He was also a corrupt Marxist, obsessed with sustaining a costly war to the north with Eritrea. Mengistu's country was starving, but the dictator had committed half of the country's GDP to military spending for an unending war over concerns that were never clarified publicly, but all about putting down insurgency.[3]

Besides the declared war with Eritrea, there were also the reckless bombings and attacks on civilians in communities thought to be protecting or supporting rebellion against the Mengistu regime. It is estimated that during the famine, much exacerbated by the dictator's policies of isolating and attacking perceived foes, Mengistu pursued a murderous campaign that killed tens of thousands of Ethiopian citizens. But there was simply nothing we could do about these atrocities. We had no choice other than focusing on the immediate needs of people who were literally starving, regardless of the factors that brought them to that terrible state of affairs.

One particularly fascinating experience turned out to be an enduring lesson about journalism. Our group was invited to witness an airdrop of grain in a remote, drought-afflicted village in the north of Ethiopia near Mekele. Importantly, we were to be accompanied by an American television press pool. The three existing networks, CBS, NBC, and ABC, agreed that there would be just one film team to capture the images that each of the networks could then cut and narrate as they wished.

All of us, the USAFA group and the TV network team, were thoroughly and simultaneously briefed by our Ethiopian security team/ minders about what to expect: A British cargo plane from the Royal Air Force would fly low over a field on the outskirts of the village and drop 50-kilogram canvas sacks of grain from the cargo bay. The sacks were expected to break open when they hit the ground so no one individual could run off with a full sack.

We were taken by helicopter to the site and stood on the field, along with villagers anxious to receive the relief supplies. Everything went exactly as we had been briefed: a flawless airdrop of an emergency grain supply, sacks bursting open, and villagers rushing out to scoop up what they could. A single, somewhat older gentlemen in a military uniform, carrying an old carbine slung over his shoulder, appeared to be overseeing the whole event, perhaps assigned to maintain civil order.

At one point the soldier raced over to a cluster of villagers arguing about a particular pile of grain apparently claimed by two factions. Rifle still on his shoulder, he dispersed the group without incident. Meanwhile the pool photographer captured all of it on film, from the arriving cargo plane to the clearing of all the grain from the field. When we returned to Addis Ababa, the raw film was sent to a production studio in Nairobi, Kenya, where each of the networks was provided a venue and equipment to cut their stories.

A few days later, on our return back to the United States with a stopover in Nairobi, Harry let us know that we were invited to see the three network stories that had run on U.S. television. Were we interested? Of course! Roll the tape. . . .

We couldn't believe what we saw. One network focused critically on the canvas bag that had burst on the field—precisely as planned, exactly as we all heard *as a group* in the briefing—characterizing it as the delivery of relief supplies in defective sacks! The second story was reasonably and objectively consistent with what actually transpired. But the third story dwelled on the hunched over soldier, carrying his ancient carbine, breaking up a grain dispute. Here's evidence, the reporter said over the video, that the Ethiopian military was trying to stop outside relief efforts.

We were almost speechless, except we were laughing at the absurdity of the three different stories, made from the same raw footage, giving three distinct versions of a simple event we had all witnessed firsthand. Before that moment, in the pre-pre-digital age, I would have considered anything on film or videotape to be unalterable reality as presented by the media. Since that moment, I look at any news story, even if documented by a photo or video, with a different understanding of what can be so easily manipulated to create an impression that may or not be real or accurate.

Both Lloyd and I were invited to join the USAFA board of directors. The following year I was asked to join the organization as a full-time senior staffer. My job would be to create a process for evaluating the hundreds of requests we were getting from organizations anxious to respond to the crisis with funds raised by "We Are the World." I was totally excited by this challenge, but I insisted on opening an East Coast satellite office. There was some reluctance initially, but the board eventually agreed; I identified office space in upper Manhattan, and Karen found a home for the family in New Rochelle, a suburb just north of the city. Working in New York allowed me to have access to my team of expert advisers, many of whom were based at Columbia University, as well as giving us proximity to the key UN organizations and the headquarters of many international relief agencies.

Board meetings—which I regularly attended at the Hollywood offices of USAFA—were always interesting and often entertaining. The meetings were interesting because these were generally smart, mostly committed people who truly wanted to do the right thing to help people caught up in an enormous ongoing humanitarian crisis. They were entertaining because, while well meaning, some of the board members were living, shall we say, the sheltered life of A-list stars. And because it was Hollywood, the trappings of fame and the perceptions of privilege seemed to be more exaggerated, even cartoonish, compared to New York.

At one meeting, a celebrity board member asked why the emergency supplies couldn't just be delivered to "the port of Africa." Belafonte patiently explained that Africa was a big continent containing more than fifty countries and that many of those nations actually had shipping ports; that there wasn't a single, generic port for the continent.

The most bizarre experience, by far, amid the strange alchemy of relief and public health professionals, business types, and global superstars also happened at a board meeting, held at the offices of Hollywood agent Ken Kragen, one of USAFA's masterminds and its board chairman. Ken had informed us that Michael Jackson was intending to show up for the next board meeting. This was a big deal, even for the Hollywood players who were in their element. Jackson was so iconic and disconnected to all but those who knew him well, that his anticipated attendance at a "business meeting" was notable.

What drew Michael to this meeting was his concern about USAFA's second major initiative, then in the early stages of planning.

The next project was concocted partly because of pushback from some in the public—and in the media—over the fact that everything raised by "We Are the World" went to Africa and nothing was designated to address serious social and economic challenges here in the United States.

So a decision was made to plan a major national initiative, called Hands Across America, designed to raise money directed toward eliminating or reducing hunger in America. The main idea was an attempt to create a single line of Americans, hand in hand, across the Continental United States. This was targeted to happen on Sunday, May 25, 1986. With celebrity endorsements and a great deal of media attention, corporate and individual donations would eventually reach some $30 million, far less than originally hoped for. (It's worth mentioning that the organization was dogged by allegations in the *New York Times* and other outlets that less than half the money raised by Hands Across America actually reached antihunger programs.) Still, it was a sincere effort to address the heartfelt public hope that the organization and the stars who were part of the effort would do something to address social and economic problems in the United States.

At the meeting in Kragen's office, Michael Jackson was laser-focused on one issue in particular: the proposed Hands Across America theme song. Kragen and Rogol had actually commissioned an advertising agency to create what they hoped would be a "catchy and heartfelt" tune to give some zest and uniqueness to the new effort. Jackson found out and was distressed, now intent on letting the board know exactly how he felt about the matter.

The long narrow table in Kragen's conference room was almost filled by USAFA board and senior staff members. Ken was at the head of the table near the window at the far end of the room. I took a seat on the long side of the table, far from the chairman's position, and immediately noticed something interesting. The only available seat now would be directly across from me. Before I had too much time to contemplate that, Michael's portly, all-business lawyer stepped into the room followed by Michael, who went directly to the empty chair opposite me. I remember no spoken greeting from Michael—just an odd grin accompanied by nodding to everyone, and no one, around the table.

Kragen, chairing the meeting, announced that he would dispense with the normal order of a typical board meeting and go right to Michael. The superstar's fingers trembled, and he seemed to be glaring at Ken Kragen as he gripped the boardroom table. An awkward silence descended. Apparently, the biggest star in the world was angry—at us.

Tears were running down the superstar's face, as Jackson let us know that God had communicated to him through his fingers when he wrote "We Are the World." Why would we even consider allowing some Madison Avenue hack to write the song for our next big venture?

The scene was beyond surreal, and I just couldn't take my eyes off Michael. This was the age before digital anything and, needless to say, I had no camera or I would have tried to capture this very, very strange scene. The best I could do, in spite of zero artistic talent, was try to subtly draw the look and feel of this moment; I wanted to remember, to capture this complex image of what seemed to me a somewhat disturbed artistic genius. There was also something profoundly sad about the scene, though I have no idea whether others in the room shared these feelings.

It is undeniable that USAFA made significant contributions to the relief effort in Africa and did so in close collaboration with UN entities and NGOs (nongovernmental organizations). But it was a struggle. For one thing, the board of USAFA had a great deal to learn, not just about relief work, but also a fundamental understanding of the continent of Africa, not to mention the nuances of the famine crisis. In spite of the glitter and utter weirdness of this massive celebrity-driven initiative, however, the motives were good—and the work, for the most part, taken very seriously. The world's oldest and largest relief organizations, from the United Nations to World Vision, Save the Children, and so many others, were working night and day to save lives, and USA for Africa was in the mix bringing assets and creativity.

Still, reflecting on the emergence of USA for Africa in 1985, it is not difficult to understand the challenges faced by this upstart, mission-driven, celebrity-studded enterprise. This was an ad hoc effort without the institutional background or experience to help figure out what to do in a deadly crisis when starvation and disease were killing thousands of people every day. Making matters worse, of course, were intractable political problems and profound resource deprivation throughout the region. On many levels, USAFA was successful, in part because the effort was not encumbered by "old ways of thinking." We were able to assimilate what worked and what didn't from the veteran organizations. We could be creative and assertive in establishing new ways of getting complex tasks accomplished. Yes, USA for Africa was starting from scratch, but it was motivated, filled with the best of intentions, and undeniably "a fast learner."

Most importantly, the multiple A-list celebrity involvement in the creation, production, recording, and marketing of the emotionally moving and commercially successful song "We Are the World" provided unprecedented access to virtually anyone in the established political or relief organizations crucial to the fight for survival in famine-affected regions of Africa. Even officials in the most staid and officious organizations were starstruck by USAFA and its impact on popular culture. It isn't fair, of course, but doors opened for us when we needed access to makers and shakers within the world of major humanitarian organizations just because this was the charity of Michael Jackson, Harry Belafonte, Kenny Rogers, and Lionel Richie.

One could—and many did—make the case that USA for Africa was not remotely ready for prime time. While most of the $50–60 million raised from the song was put to good use, the process was not without serious problems. By the end of 1985, the press was clamoring for accountability. Where did the money actually go? Were lives saved? Why was it taking so long to get the money distributed while children were dying of hunger?

Desperate to get money out the door, USA for Africa lost its cool under the glaring spotlight of media scrutiny and succumbed to the pressure. As director of grants for USA for Africa, I had established a number of expert advisory groups to help sift through and rate the hundreds of applications we were receiving, carefully evaluating which groups actually had the capacity and experience to make effective and timely use of a grant from us.

There were many potential grants and relationships that my advisory teams and I rejected as questionable or risky investments. One request denial was to a private company in Great Britain that requested funding to provide spare tires needed for relief trucks in targeted countries. That company had been accused of fraudulent practices, and its CEO was later investigated for such. The second grant I had great issue with was a $5.2 million appropriation to an African bank that already had a reputation for shady dealings and could provide no assurance that it would be sufficiently accountable for how a USAFA grant would be spent. In December of 1985, with press pressure mounting to "move the money" to Africa, USAFA's board, over my strenuous objections, pushed out the funds to both of the two questionable organizations.

The problems were deeper than a disagreement over how those funding decisions were being made. The bigger issue was that I was seen by virtually everyone else in the USAFA leadership as pretty much "off the reservation," by virtue of geography but, more importantly, attitude. The whole situation didn't end particularly well for me. My departure from USAFA was strange and gradual, starting with my not being included on the board's new executive committee, a subgroup of the board abruptly assigned responsibility for all major decision making.

If nothing else, USAFA was committed to making sure that no hint of internal turmoil would ever leak. There was never any kind of public statement, but I became persona non grata, no longer at the table when and where significant decisions were being made. The bottom line was that—no fuss, no muss—the matter of Irwin Redlener, general troublemaker from the other coast, was "handled." I was disappointed, feeling righteous and offended, but the truth is that I was also impressed by the clean slicing and dicing these Hollywood people were so good at.

Still, at least in retrospect, the experience of working with and for USAFA was a major opportunity for me to participate in an effort of enormous scope, collaborating with people and agencies driven by a mission, even as they were so often cuffed and dulled by immovable bureaucracies. Overall, it would be ludicrous to conclude that the impact of this entire effort was anything other than spectacular, my own personal experiences notwithstanding. These megastars stepped up to make a difference in a true global catastrophe. Was it perfect? Of course not—but neither are many efforts made by some of the most experienced relief organizations on the planet.

As was the case for Bob Geldorf's extraordinary Live Aid project, USAFA's success wasn't just about the money raised by these legendary stars and cultural icons of the 1980s. It was also very much about the sincerity of their efforts and their unparalleled ability to raise global awareness around one of the worst human tragedies of the twentieth century.

In another moment of pure serendipity, in November 1986 I had come out to Los Angeles for a board meeting and was standing in Marty Rogol's office when he got a call from one of the "We Are the World" singers. The superstar wanted to know if any of the money raised could be used to help the growing problem of homelessness in New York City. Marty was pushing back, reminding him that we were committed to spending the money for African famine relief.

"But maybe you should meet with our director of grants, Dr. Irwin Redlener," I heard Marty say. "He's based in New York and might be a good person to touch base with."

And that's how, just a few weeks later, I met Paul Simon and took him for a tour of New York City's hellish welfare hotels for homeless families.

Homeless Children, Limousines, and the Birth of the Children's Health Fund

The plan was for Paul Simon to pick me up at the New York offices of USAFA. I didn't know what to expect or how this day was going to go, but I wasn't surprised when it started out in rock-star style as his late-model chauffeured limo pulled up in front of my building. Paul and his friend and publicist, Dan Klores, were in the backseat, so I climbed into the auxiliary row facing the two of them. Paul and Dan were friendly enough to me and interested in where we were going, though with Paul's magnificent *Graceland* tour pending, they had business to discuss.

The first stop was the headquarters of the Association to Benefit Children (ABC), a program focused on caring for children afflicted with HIV/AIDS acquired at birth from infected mothers. Gretchen Buchenholz, ABC's dynamic director, was waiting for us at the organization's Upper East Side headquarters. Gretchen was anxious to talk about ABC and introduced us to some of the children, including a three-year-old Hispanic girl who was not doing well. She would not make eye contact with us and was not interested in speaking. Gretchen told us that she was generally bright and communicative but had a particularly poor prognosis; in essence, she was not expected to survive another six months.

Gretchen joined us for the ride over to the Martinique Hotel, one of the facilities that the city was using to "warehouse" homeless families. Along the way, she gave us a crash course in city politics and the attempts to manage a rapidly growing homeless family population in New York.

Beginning the early 1980s, New York mayor Ed Koch faced a major crisis as the prevalence of homelessness among families was rising dramatically. By 1986, as a result of many factors, including a shortage of affordable housing for low-income residents in the city, some 4,000 families with more than 10,000 children found themselves with no resources and no place to live.[4] The city needed to provide shelter, and the Koch administration had no choice but to find accommodations, somewhere, somehow. Thousands of people needed a roof over their heads, and not just for a few days or a couple of weeks until a new apartment placement became available. There was hardly anything "available," ever. As a result, the city was placing these forgotten families in congregate shelters and privately owned, very run-down "welfare hotels" for stays that averaged eighteen months to two years. The Martinique was the biggest and most infamous welfare hotel in the city, the San Quentin of shelters. Our visit there powerfully confirmed that the conditions in this squalid, surreal last stop for the city's most under-resourced families deserved its awful reputation.

And it wasn't just the welfare hotels. Thousands of homeless singles and families stayed in enormous open spaces in New York's armories; cots and cribs crammed together, some occupied by young families with babies and toddlers, others by homeless, alcoholic men with histories of mental illness. Assignments in the armories frequently lasting as long as eighteen months.

Having worked in rural Honduras, Guatemala, and Lee County, Arkansas, and having seen the ravages of famine in Africa, I was no stranger to suffering children. But none of us was prepared for what we saw and heard when we walked through the front door of the once stately hotel on the corner of Broadway and Thirty-First Street. This was extreme poverty and deprivation in the very heart of one of the world's great cities, a center of global media, great wealth, and innovation. Everyone knew that New York, like any other major metropolis, had communities of poverty. Neighborhoods in Harlem, the South Bronx, and central Brooklyn were all struggling with serious long-standing economic and social problems. Still, the Martinique was something different: a tiny island of despair, just a short walk from Times Square and the heart of the theater district, where New Yorkers and tourists from around the world walked by the old hotel in droves, few aware of the chaos that engulfed the lives of its involuntary guests who were "checked in" because they, and the city, were simply out of options.

As soon as we were inside the main lobby, I remember thinking that something was terribly wrong. Homeless families, crying children, and security guards filled the lobby. Tough guys with disheveled suits were glaring at us from windowed offices overlooking the once stately check-in desk. Gretchen made the first move, introducing us to the man who seemed to be the manager, explaining why Paul, the singer-songwriter legend, was standing in his lobby. After an awkward moment or two of questioning, he agreed to let us walk up to the hotel's mezzanine.

The place was teeming with children; hundreds of kids and their families were being warehoused in this seventeen-story building which clearly should have been condemned for a multitude of building code violations, from peeling paint and broken electrical outlets to mouse droppings, nonworking elevators, and broken plumbing. We would eventually learn that prostitution and a thriving illegal drug trade were business as usual in the hotel.

The scene on the mezzanine, which had some forty desks occupied by workers from multiple city and voluntary agencies, including ABC, was a cacophony of babies crying, parents pleading, workers explaining, and hotel security personnel scowling. Gretchen explained, "This is where the residents get information about available services, but most of these people just want to get out of here. Can't say that I blame them."

Around the corner on the mezzanine level was the entry to the old ballroom, where we saw a long line of children and their parents snaking down the corridor. "What's going on here?" I asked. A staff person from one of the agencies said, "The Coalition for the Homeless distributes hot food once a day up here. And for many children, this might well be their only meal of the day."

Gretchen offered to take us to the fourteenth floor to see some of the conditions in the actual rooms. Paul was mostly quiet but focused, asking me questions as we walked through the hotel: "Why are these people here?" or "Why are there so many children?" and "What help are they getting?"

A number of mothers told us that their children were rarely able to see a doctor, that treks to the emergency rooms were arduous, long, and chaotic—intolerable unless their child was really sick. Regular access to doctors for immunizations, checkups, and health screenings was virtually out of the question. Gretchen confirmed all of this and more—and happened to mention that she and her staff were considering using a mobile unit to set up a childhood vaccination service for homeless children.

This registered with me as a very intriguing concept. I was reminded of the house calls I had made nearly every day in rural Arkansas. We visited homebound patients where they lived, not expecting them to make the trip to our clinic. Why not find a way to do the same for homeless children in New York? Instead of traveling into the backwoods of the Delta with an assistant and little black bag of medical supplies in an old government surplus Jeep, what if we brought the whole medical team in a fully equipped mobile clinic *to them*? I kept thinking about this idea and was ready to discuss it with Paul when we spoke a few days after our visit to the Martinique. He had been as shocked as I was to see the conditions in the hotel and was interested to know what I thought we could do. I obliged him with a description of a new program to get medical care to children in the shelters: we would create a state-of-the-art, rolling pediatric clinic staffed by a full medical team.

I had no idea how Paul would respond to my idea about a mobile clinic for homeless children in New York City—and whether he was still interested on any level. Would he be interested in helping me create a rolling pediatric clinic?

But my anxiety was short-lived; Paul's reaction was immediate. "That's a great idea," he said. "Let's do it."

The next move was to describe the concept in more detail, which I did in a document dubbed "The New York Children's Health Project," the program that turned out to be the first project of the Children's Health Fund (CHF), an organization that would be brought to operational fruition within a year of that visit to the old Martinique. I had the vision down but told Paul that we needed someone to develop and implement a workable plan—and I also happened to know just the right person for the job. I explained all this to Paul. He thought for a moment before responding. He was taking it all in and, I guessed, trying to process how an undertaking like this would or would not affect his immediate plans for the *Graceland* tour.

"Who do you have in mind?" asked Paul.

"Karen Redlener," I said. "My wife."

"Maybe so," Paul replied. "How do we know if she'll do it? Have you asked her?"

"Not really. Let's take her out to dinner and present the idea," I suggested. Paul agreed.

Karen is a smart, experienced health care administrator and innovator who had been working with me since she joined our VISTA project in Arkansas, where, as a twenty-one-year-old recently minted Pomona College graduate, she was an unstoppable force in developing essential programs for many children in East Arkansas. She single-handedly developed a social services program for the clinic and screened nearly one thousand rural poor children for hearing, vision, and developmental problems. Later, when we moved to Miami, she organized another screening program at a University of Miami children and youth clinic and coordinated mental health services for the Dade County Head Start Program.

In Utica, Karen helped set up my pediatric practice and continued her long-standing connection with Head Start by serving on their local advisory board. There was no doubt in my mind that this idea for a new way to get health care to homeless children in New York City would be perfectly consistent with Karen's interests and skills. Translating the idea into a working program would be a job I thought she would relish. At the time, however, Karen wanted to go to graduate school, and I shouldn't have been so sure about how she would react to the idea of taking on this program development full-time—especially right now.

Paul chose a local favorite restaurant around the corner from his Upper West Side Manhattan apartment. We met there at a little after 8:00 one fall evening. At first, there was just small talk about the new album and plans for the *Graceland* tour. But Paul wanted to know more about us: Where did we grow up? What was it like working together in Arkansas? What about our own children? He couldn't have been more relaxed or engaged in the conversation.

Then, down to business.

Karen had gotten a preview about our agenda prior to dinner, reacting in a way that was tough to read. At dinner, Paul led the way in describing what we were thinking about. I was pleasantly surprised at how well he was able to describe the concept. I chimed in with details.

Karen was initially ambivalent about taking on the project. The past few years had been spent mostly at home raising four children. Now she had finally found the opportunity to go back to school to fulfill a longtime goal, getting a master's degree. "I don't know," she said to Paul. "I am finally in grad school, and it's important to me."

Paul said, "I understand."

Bad answer, I thought. We would have to push Karen to take this on—and I knew her soft spots.

167

"Listen," I said, "we can provide health care to hundreds—maybe thousands—of homeless kids. Most have never even seen a doctor outside of an emergency room."

That got her attention. Paul pulled back, just listening to the conversation unfold between Karen and me. I continued, "Karen, you get what these kids need. We've seen it before back in Lee County. These children in the shelters are under-immunized. A lot of them have hearing loss and speech and language delays from ear infections that were never treated right from the beginning. Asthma is epidemic in the shelters—and so are nutrition deficits and emotional problems." I could tell it was sinking in; she was listening carefully—and so was Paul.

At the right moment, Paul added the clincher:

"Karen, these kids need this program—and Irwin says *we can't do it without you.*"

She looked at Paul, then me.

"I get it. And I think I can do it," she told us.

Paul, soon to be leaving on his *Graceland* world tour, offered Karen his office in the fabled Brill Building just north of Times Square at Forty-Ninth and Broadway—probably the most prestigious address in New York City for music professionals. Music legends like Cab Calloway, Nat King Cole, Duke Ellington, Carole King, Marvin Hamlisch—and Paul Simon—had composed hit after hit from offices in the eleven-story Art Deco institution, once described as a vertical Tin Pan Alley. At Paul's desk in his fifth-floor office, surrounded by music memorabilia from Paul's more than thirty years in the industry, Karen worked to convert the concept of the New York Children's Health Project into an action plan. There was much to be done, connecting with a multitude of city agencies and community-based organizations, figuring out which community-based organizations were working in the shelters, designing our first mobile clinic, and so on.

Karen had no model to emulate and began with a blank sheet of paper. In 1986 there were mobile units used for health screening, health education, and childhood vaccinations. But putting a fully operational pediatric office on wheels? There was just no precedent we were aware of. We would need room for doctors and nurses and all the equipment of a modern doctor's office stuffed into a facility that could move to several locations every day.

We also had to educate ourselves on the situation regarding homeless children and available health care in the city. We didn't want to duplicate services, but it quickly became clear that ours would be a unique system that would fill a desperately needed gap in medical care for the homeless.

Although anybody should have seen that the need for this service was urgent, we faced a decidedly mixed reaction.

On the one hand, then Manhattan Borough President David Dinkins—the future mayor—was immediately receptive. Paul and I requested an appointment to see him, and his staff responded right away. Dinkins had—and still has—a special affinity for children. As borough president and then New York City mayor, Dinkins always prioritized programs and resources for children. On the other hand, the reaction from Mayor Ed Koch and his administration was an entirely different story. The Koch administration had deliberately designed the homeless shelter system so that a family would be assigned to a facility as far as possible from their original neighborhood. The idea was to keep families from becoming "too comfortable" in the shelter system. But this arrangement also forced people to sever critical ties to their support system, including any doctors and specialists their children might have been seeing for, say, the management of serious chronic conditions like congenital heart disease or long-standing anemia.

Clearly, the New York City mayor's office did not want to recognize there was a major problem with homeless children's access to regular medical care, and even if there were a crisis, it could and should be addressed by city agencies—no need for the kind of nongovernmental strategy Paul and I were bringing to the table. We realized that to administration officials, support for our program might be interpreted to mean that the city wasn't doing its job! There was, in fact, some truth to that interpretation.

In meetings and phone calls with people in Koch's office and relevant city agencies, they insisted that our mobile clinic idea was superficial and not helpful. We protested, saying that more than 10,000 children were living in homeless shelters and they weren't getting the health care they needed.

"I don't believe your data," one city official told me in a meeting.

"It's *your* data," I responded.

She changed the subject.

"Whatever the number of children, we have plenty of free health care clinics in New York for people to go to."

She was wrong, and we had the evidence to prove it.

Other than David Dinkins, when he served as mayor in the early 1990s, this hostile attitude from city officials persisted for more than two decades. Mayor Rudy Giuliani, generally shortsighted, petty, and vengeful, was a disaster when it came to addressing the problem of homelessness.

We were actively speaking out about the epidemic of asthma among homeless children and had proposed an innovative new program to get this situation under control. But when the City Council passed a budget appropriation providing money for a children's asthma program, the mayor's people delayed the start-up of the program, burying the actual distribution of the appropriated funds under a virtual mountain of administrative nonsense.

At one point, I was quoted in the New York *Daily News* as being frustrated by the unending delays in getting the program started. Asthma was an epidemic in the shelters, with more than one in three children having active symptoms from undiagnosed or inadequately treated asthma.

Giuliani, offended that I had called him out publicly, shot back at a press conference:

"Redlener thinks that he and his programs are like 'sacred cows.' Well, we're going to make hamburger meat out of him."

Raising objections to our new program was not limited to city officials. Surprisingly, homeless advocates, and even other doctors who I assumed would be helpful, offered little support, essentially implying that we were inappropriately stepping on and into *their* turf. Even my fellow pediatricians listened politely and then assured us they were working on the problems of health care for homeless children. "Even if you do decide to do this," one colleague told me, "you don't have the experience."

One prominent academic pediatrician assured me, "The problem of access to quality health care for homeless kids is under control. We're taking care of it." Interesting, I thought, but I knew that nothing could be further from the truth.

Many homeless advocates clearly resented Paul. They viewed him as an outsider who had no business even talking about homelessness and children.

In one meeting at my new Manhattan offices, one furious activist for the poor said, "Who does Paul Simon think he is? What right does he have to come in here like he knows everything? He knows *nothing*."

I was glad Paul wasn't there to hear this noise.

What these long-struggling advocates actually disliked was the fact that this famous musician would bring a lot of attention to homelessness, when they had been laboring for years with little recognition and few resources.

People tend to think that there is some kind of "kumbaya" collaboration among nonprofits working with the poor. Actually, the politics of interorganizational relationships are far more complicated than people think. In reality, there is intense competition among nonprofits as they try to elbow each other out for funds, attention, and resources. Media attention and celebrity support really bring out the bitterness.

Undaunted by the persistent skepticism and hostility, Karen hammered away, determined to get a mobile clinic built and on the road. Within three months, she designed the first unit—two fully equipped examination rooms, a bathroom, a nurse's station, and a waiting area—all squeezed into a thirty-foot-long, fully self-contained clinic on wheels. The cost to build that first unit in 1986 was $85,000—a fraction of the $300,000 it would cost in 2015. On top of the construction costs, funds would be required to staff and operate the program, which we estimated would amount to at least $500,000 a year. At that point, it wasn't clear who would raise the money or how. Paul Simon volunteered to reach out to his friends in the music business for support of the new program.

In his office, I heard him on the phone talking to one of his show business friends, trying to cajole a donation. He was clearly having a hard time.

"No, it would not be *in* a clinic. It would be in a clinic in a *bus*," Paul said.

He listened as his clearly skeptical would-be donor asked some questions.

"We need $85,000 just to build the mobile clinic," he said.

He listened to the response. By his expression, I could tell it wasn't going well.

"No, that won't pay for operating it," he said. "That's just to *build* it."

The call was over, and Paul was frustrated.

A few days later, Paul called me to talk about the fund-raising efforts. Clearly, the skepticism we faced went beyond homeless advocates and the mayor's office. Private donors weren't buying it either. I was growing concerned that we had a great concept but would have no funds to carry it forward.

"How is it going?" I asked.

There was a short silence, then Paul said, "Not good. This is a lot more difficult than I expected."

"I was afraid of that," I replied.

It was indeed frustrating. We had documented the needs, we had developed a plan to address them, and we had a manufacturer.

This was very real to us. But others couldn't see it—at least not yet.

"You know what?" said Paul suddenly. "I'm just going to pay for it myself."

Clearly, he had been thinking about this.

I wouldn't have blamed him for giving up. He had tried hard, and we were grateful for all his efforts.

But now his offer changed everything.

Paul's generosity would pay off on other fronts, too. With the funding to build the mobile clinic secure, New York Hospital–Cornell Medical Center agreed to sponsor the program. At least initially, the department of pediatrics at the staid Upper East Side hospital that mostly catered to high-end, affluent patients reacted with great enthusiasm, certainly intrigued by my partnership with Paul Simon. He was a big catch for an institution that really liked the public visibility that came with caring for and relating to the rich and famous.

Housing the new program at Cornell's medical center was beneficial to us as well. It represented a link to a prestigious medical institution, giving us instant credibility. I was appointed the hospital's chief of outpatient pediatrics and an associate professor in the medical school. By July 1987 we had moved our offices to New York–Cornell's campus on East Sixty-Eighth Street, ordered the mobile clinic, and hired staff. This was big. We were about to launch a program that would provide high-quality medical care to some of the most disenfranchised children in America. We knew that the first stop for this new mobile clinic would be to care for the children in the Martinique Hotel.

The mobile clinic finally arrived in September 1987. On that early fall day, Karen and I stood on the corner a block east of York Avenue and Sixty-Eighth Street, waiting for the unit, driven in from its Midwest manufacturer, to turn the corner from York Avenue and trundle down the street toward us. For more than a year, all of us—Paul, Karen, and I—had been working to make this day materialize, and any minute we'd get our first look at the pediatric mobile clinic that had heretofore existed only in our imaginations.

When the mobile clinic appeared at the back door of the pediatric clinic, we were totally blown away. With its sleek body and wraparound windshield, it was part bus, part RV—and, to us, totally beautiful.

And blue. *Blue?* We had ordered clinical white, with an accent stripe in blue. For a split second, we looked at each other and stared back at the mobile clinic now parked, motor still running, on the street in front of us. Then we realized that the color was actually perfect—a gorgeous shade of vibrant blue that became the norm for the dozens of units that would become part of CHF's fleet in the years to come. This was a mistake that turned into an asset that truly stood the test of time.

Six weeks later, on a cold, drizzly early morning in November 1987, the new medical team and I boarded the bus for its maiden "house call." Steve Diaz, our newly hired driver, guided the vehicle south toward the Martinique, forty blocks away through choking Manhattan rush hour traffic. It was the biggest vehicle Steve, a former auto mechanic, had ever driven, and he maneuvered the thirty-foot-long vehicle carefully as the usual honking taxicabs and city buses swerved in front of us. Along with Steve and me, nurse-practitioner Andrea Berne and registrar Ruth Hedley were on board. Steve and Ruth stayed on the job, growing with CHF for thirty years!

Thanksgiving of 1987 was fast approaching, but the future for some ten thousand homeless children and their families in the city wasn't about holiday festivities and tables full of plentiful food in warm, inviting homes. This was, and is, like so many other places in the United States, a city of stark contrasts, and the new mobile clinic was headed toward a place where hopelessness and unending need were a sad reality for lots of struggling families. But, as I found so often in the coming years, in spite of what they didn't have, many of these children still managed to hold onto dreams and aspirations that sustained them through the adversities over which they had little control.

As we approached the Martinique, we saw at least forty mothers, fathers, and children already lined up against the outside wall of the dilapidated building. We no idea what kind of reception we would be getting, and we were genuinely surprised to see so many people waiting for us. Word was out that we would be there to provide free medical care to children who were staying in the hotel. How and what that meant was a bit unclear for the families, and for us, too. We had the mission and the model, but just how it would all work on the street remained to be seen.

By 9:30, we were seeing our first patients. Steve—now functioning as security guard, patient coordinator, and all-a round positive presence—was making his way down the line greeting each family, making a list of children who would be seeing the new doctor and his team. One after another, children climbed on board with their parents. We treated ear infections, asthma, impetigo, lice, intestinal infections, and gave needed immunizations. We assessed children—and their parents—who seemed depressed and anxious, traumatized by the experience of being homeless, with no way to escape the ugliness and chaos of the Martinique.

Many experiences I had while working in the mobile clinics caring for highly vulnerable homeless children in New York reminded me of the situations we had faced in Lee County some fourteen years earlier, and, for that matter, the realities of overt child poverty in Miami. The children who were being sheltered in the Martinique had the same look of despair and poverty as did children in the Arkansas Delta or downtown Miami. I was in America's largest city, far from the cotton fields and overt racism of rural Arkansas, but witnessing yet another terrible injustice that was taking a palpable toll on children. I wondered, what had changed in America? Were we "winning" what President Lyndon Johnson declared as a "War on Poverty"? From what I saw in that new mobile pediatric unit caring for children of the Martinique, there might well be a war on—but poverty was winning.

CHF hit the New York scene in a high-visibility celebrity spotlight. The vibe was exhilarating, reinforced just two months after we began the program by a front-page story in the *New York Times*. Among other reactions, that story prompted a call from a lawyer I had never heard of. Bobby Tannenhauser had read the *Times* story and tracked me down that very day.

"Hello. Is this Irwin Redlener, the pediatrician?"

"Yes. Who's this?"

"You don't know me. The name's Bob Tannenhauser, and I am a lawyer in New York."

"Okay," I responded. "What can I do for you?"

"What can *you* do for *me*? You mean how can *I* help *you*! What do you need?"

I thought for a moment.

"Well, I wish you were a pediatrician, but there is something I could use legal assistance with. We're hearing from a lot of folks who want to contribute to our new program, and I'd rather not have the funds come through my hospital. Would you consider helping us establish a formal, separate identity as a charitable organization?"

Bobby responded without so much as a pause to think about it, "Yes, of course. Let's meet and talk about it."

This would be just what we needed. CHF's connection with New York Hospital, situated in New York's affluent an Upper East Side, was fraught, mostly because of noncompatible missions of the academic medical center and our new program. New York Hospital was preoccupied with its reputation as "the place to go" for the rich and well-known. Hospital leaders, initially thrilled with the Paul Simon connection, were growing increasingly ambivalent about our well-publicized focus on homeless children, not exactly consistent with their commitment to a decidedly more affluent patient population. The honeymoon was over.

The meeting with Bobby happened three days later. Within a week he initiated the process necessary to create the official tax-exempt, not-for-profit status of our new organization. There was more: Bobby gave us space in his law office as CHF's new "headquarters." Then it was just a matter of time before Bobby, his wife Carol, Karen, and I became close friends as we chartered the course of what would be an enduring, innovative health care program for some of America's most disadvantaged children.

By the middle of 1989, I had grown significantly anxious about mission incompatibility with New York Hospital. Sharing my concerns with Karen, she agreed that our expanding work with homeless children would not be tolerated there for long, so neither of us was all that surprised when our concerns were borne out in a confrontation with the pediatric department chairperson. We had strong evidence that funds being raised for the mobile child health program were being shifted out of our budget to other academic needs. So, in the summer of 1990, we moved our program to Montefiore Hospital in the Bronx, where the institution's mission was very much about serving the underserved and where we were welcomed with open arms.

Meeting the Tannenhausers was not the only positive outcome from the *Times* article. *Today Show* host Jane Pauley and her husband Garry Trudeau, famed political cartoonist and creator of *Doonesbury*, saw the article the morning it came out. Just by chance, a week earlier, Paul and I had written to Jane to see if she would be interested in what we were trying to do for New York's homeless children. I didn't know her personally but had always been impressed with how she expressed herself on television, clearly a caring and compassionate person.

Jane's response to our letter and the *Times* article was enthusiastic, and she clearly understood what we were trying to accomplish. She wanted to be involved—and we couldn't have been more excited to hear that. Thirty years later, Jane has proven herself to be one of CHF's longest standing and most influential board members.

More press was coming. A few weeks after the *Times* front-pager, *Newsweek* magazine published a two-page spread about our program. I must say that this rush of early press seemed a bit premature, but I understood why it was happening. Paul's celebrity was irresistible to the press and the public. Paul was not only experiencing extraordinary reviews for his new *Graceland* album and selling out concerts around the world, he was also in the news.

With the release of *Graceland*, a beautiful, barrier-busting artistic achievement, Paul faced intense, unexpected criticism, primarily from the highly political South African antiapartheid party, the African National Congress. But it wasn't just the ANC leadership that went after him. Musicians and artists around the world had declared a cultural boycott of South Africa, vowing never to perform in that country until apartheid ended. Many of Paul's peer performers joined in the criticism.

But for Paul and so many others, this was different. Apartheid was suppressing the artistry and careers of black South African musical artists and limiting the possibility for other black African performers to achieve success. Paul went to South Africa to hear, create, and record with the very artists who were being suppressed by the apartheid government. Paul found tremendous talents and gave them opportunities to be heard around the world.

Looking back at the controversy, Paul had no regrets for how *Graceland* came about and what it did for the global exposure to extraordinary African music. He was quoted in an article by journalist Robert Denselow in April 2012: "Personally, I feel I'm with the musicians," he said. "I'm with the artists. I didn't ask the permission of the ANC. I didn't ask permission of Buthelezi, or Desmond Tutu, or the Pretoria government. And to tell you the truth, I have a feeling that when there are radical transfers of power on either the left or the right, the artists always get screwed. The guys with the guns say, 'This is important,' and the guys with guitars don't have a chance."[5]

Meanwhile, as Karen was working on mobile unit design in Paul's office, many other U.S. cities were reporting upsurges in family homelessness. With our program getting lots of national media attention, we were fielding scores of inquiries from across the country—including from rural towns wallowing in poverty, so very reminiscent of where Karen and I found each other and discovered a shared mission in Lee County. Desperate community leaders inquired about our new initiative, asking if they could somehow get a mobile clinic in their own communities. If the needs were legitimate and a mobile clinic could be part of the solution, we would do everything we could to help wherever it made sense.

But the real solutions to health care challenges related to homelessness and poverty were not going to be solved by fifty, or five thousand, pediatric mobile units. Big solutions could only come with significant support from government, especially at the federal level. What could make a difference might be a concerted, full-blown advocacy agenda. We would be the doctors taking care of children in great need, but we would also do whatever it took to wake up the public—and especially elected officials—to what we were dealing with. In essence, we were picking at the edges of a problem of massive scale and scope.

There was never a question of how we were going to approach caring for the children who were depending on us to give them the best possible medical attention. But I was more than aware that none of this would be sustainable unless we had the necessary resources to pay the staff, maintain the mobile clinics, and set up a rigorous advocacy program. I wasn't exactly sure where the money was going to come from or how we would sustain public interest in the plight and challenges faced by homeless and indigent families who wanted nothing more than some assurance that their children would have a decent shot at getting and staying healthy.

The plan was that we would strive to provide gold-standard medical care for every child we saw, every day, at every site our mobile units visited. Every parent would be treated with the respect that he or she deserved but rarely got. We saw—and still see—all children filled with unrealized promise. Our job was to make sure that no health problems stood in the way of children's chance to realize their potential. But more than that, we committed to making sure that the nonmedical issues that needed attention, from housing and Medicaid assistance to school enrollment, were actively included in our very expansive sense of what doctors who care for poor children need to keep front of mind.

All that was clear from the outset. Explicitly recognized in CHF's original mission was the simple fact that we would not be satisfied with—or settle for—just being really good doctors. Our whole team—and everyone that ever worked for us—had to understand and embrace the notion that we were not just doctors, nurses, administrators, or mobile clinic drivers. We were, individually and collectively, serious advocates for the children we served directly and for all children facing adversity who weren't getting the health care they needed. That's why I talked Paul into joining me in a couple of fascinating visits to Capitol Hill.

Traveling to Washington with Paul was, as we used to say, "a trip." Senate doors opened wide for the superstar (and me, his tagalong physician-advocate). We initially focused on the Senate and visited many offices. We sought opportunities to tell senators what we knew about homeless and disadvantaged children and the problems of getting necessary medical care. Many of our visits to powerful leaders, including Senators Jay Rockefeller, Bob Kerry, Chris Dodd, Majority Leader George Mitchell, Orin Hatch, and others from both sides of the aisle, were coordinated by one of our new friends, Steve Ricchetti, then a health care advocate working the halls of Congress. Steve went on to take a prominent role coordinating congressional liaisons in the Bill Clinton White House. Eventually Steve wound up as Vice President Joe Biden's chief of staff, remaining an important advocate in the halls of power. The Senate relationships we made between 1988 and the early 1990s were enduring and led to many other critical contacts over the years. We used this access to push for policies and legislation that would benefit children who needed more resources, more programs, and a broad focus of attention.

One important outcome of those early introductions to key senators was an opportunity in 1988 to testify before Senator Christopher Dodd's Subcommittee on Care for the Homeless. I talked about the situations we were seeing in New York City. In particular, I focused on a particular clinical problem that illustrated the consequences of homelessness for children. At the time, one of the most important medical problems faced by children in shelters was undertreated ear infections. Without good access to medical care and medications, acute infections became painful and chronic, often leading to hearing loss.

Two highly rewarding advocacy accomplishments came out of this hearing. First, we convinced Senator Dodd and his colleagues to create a special amendment to the new McKinney Act, a legislative initiative to help deal with rising homelessness in America. Our amendment created special funding for programs focused on homeless children. Success!

The second outcome of my Senate appearance was a bit more mysterious—but equally exciting. It turned out that, totally unbeknownst to me, a representative from a pharmaceutical company was in the gallery listening to the hearing. I didn't know it at the time, but the executive worked for Lederle, a long-since-gone pharma that had a commercial interest in the issue I testified about. When he got back to the company's headquarters and told colleagues about the testimony, they arranged for their PR representative to reach out to me.

"Dr. Redlener?"

"Yes"

"My name is Gloria Janata. I work for a drug company that is interested in what you had to say at Senator Dodd's hearing. They are intrigued and concerned about problems with treating ear infections in children. And they might have something that could be very helpful in managing these conditions, especially for the homeless kids you're caring for."

"What company is this, and what do they have that might be helpful to me?" I said, trying to hide my natural cynicism about a cold call like this.

"Sorry," Gloria responded. "For now, I can't reveal the name of the company. But I'll tell you this: they have a new liquid antibiotic that is highly effective for ear infections but doesn't need refrigeration and only requires a single daily dose for ten days."

She had my undivided attention. Among the challenges of treating infections in homeless children was that all of the existing antibiotics in liquid form needed to be kept cold, a major problem for many family shelters where reliable access to a working refrigerator was highly uncertain. Moreover, the lives of homeless families were riddled with constant stress and terrible pressures on parents to find permanent housing, feasible employment, and access to school for their children. Making sure that one of the children got the required three or four daily doses of antibiotics was a challenge more difficult than most economically secure families can likely imagine. So, all in all, the idea of this new once-a-day, okay-at-room-temperature antibiotic was more than a little intriguing.

"So, Ms. Gloria Janata, what do we need to do?"

"Well, I've been asked to do some 'due diligence' to confirm that you are indeed on the leading edge of providing high-quality medical care to homeless kids. In due time, I'll tell you what company I'm working for. I am sure they'll want to meet you, too."

Over the next few weeks, we worked with Gloria. She saw our programs in action, and we provided plenty of data. Before we knew it, she was hooked and revealed that she was, indeed, working for Lederle, a pharmaceutical company then owned by the multinational firm called American Cyanamid. It turned out that the new antibiotic they had developed, called Suprax, was a truly effective once-a-day drug that was stable at room temperature—perfect for what we needed. In short order we were bonding with Lederle executives, all under the watchful eye of Gloria, who was clearly trying to help make something happen for CHF. When all the pieces were in place, Gloria called.

"Hey, Irwin, great news. Lederle wants to make a major contribution to CHF."

"Terrific! What do they have in mind?"

"How about this: a cash grant of $75,000 and, get this, they plan on donating $10 million worth of Suprax! How about that?" she said. I'm sure she was expecting something more than the moment of silence I offered up as my initial response. "What's the matter?"

"Well, Gloria, I don't want to seem ungrateful. But the problem is, there is no way I can possibly use that much antibiotic. If I can be blunt with you, what I need is support for our programs. That means money to pay staff and maintain the mobile clinics." (I am sure I sounded confident and clear, but I was totally nervous that I might offend my new friend and damage the fragile sapling of our new relationship with a major pharmaceutical company.)

But Gloria's reaction was perfect.

"Look, I get it, of course. Let me bring them a different idea— and I'll get back to you."

I hung up the phone and took a slow, deep breath, just hoping I hadn't screwed this up. But the anxiety was ill-founded. Gloria called back the next week and let me know that David Bethune, Lederle's president, wanted me to join him and his executive team for lunch at the company's headquarters in New Jersey.

Some lunch it was—tasty food and good conversation. After coffee was served, Dave leaned over, took an envelope out of his jacket, and casually passed it to me.

"Listen, Dr. Redlener, we really like what you're doing and want to help make this all work. Go ahead and open that envelope."

And so I did—and discovered a check from Lederle made out to the Children's Health Fund in the amount of $1 million! I truly was overwhelmed, for a moment didn't quite know what to say. It was more than a little notable that there was no other paperwork in the envelope—no "terms," no delineation of deliverables, no timeline, no explicit requirements—just that check with six zeros. I smiled and looked around the room, turned back to David Bethune, and managed to say something that has endured as a principal tenet of relationship with every donor that has helped us since that day.

"David, I am incredibly grateful for this. I know you have not set conditions around what we will do with that money. I interpret that as trusting me and our team to do what's necessary and do it well. And I want you to know that I deeply appreciate this trust. Be assured that you will never regret this gift, and I promise you that we will over-deliver on whatever expectations you might have."

Bethune and I stood as if on cue and shook hands. I thanked him and the others in the room, and lunch was over. As I left to drive back to our offices in New York, I knew that CHF would be sustained and grow, that we were beginning an odyssey, fulfilling a mission that meant everything to me. That this epiphany happened in the aftermath of a corporate meeting, not in Washington, not even when I was doing pediatrics in the back room of a mobile clinic, was notable.

We couldn't help comparing the Lederle process with what it took to get our first local government grant. Through the good offices of then Manhattan borough president David Dinkins, the only public official in New York who believed in us, a small "token" grant of $35,000 was authorized. After reams of required paperwork were completed, the contract was submitted to the relevant city agency. We finally got the government check. It took eighteen months—ten times longer than it took Lederle to issue a million-dollar check, essentially without conditions or paperwork.

I've thought about that experience a great deal over the years. In some ways, getting huge support from Lederle in a very simple process set unrealistic expectations that every corporate grant would be similarly obtained and every CEO as trusting as Bethune. Of course, that was not to be the case. By 2004 most corporate foundations had become far more formal, much like major independent foundations process, though rarely as onerous as a government agency protocols.

With that first million dollars, I was able to implement the CHF programs that I had envisioned from the beginning, creating a model in New York that could be replicated anywhere in the country, in urban and rural communities alike. So when pediatricians in New Jersey reached out and requested a mobile unit to provide medical care to homeless children in Newark, we could—and did—say, "Of course! Let's get to work."

There was one more extraordinary experience in those early years. In December 1987, not long after we started seeing children in the Martinique, Paul Simon hosted an enormous concert at Madison Square Garden. Through Paul's efforts, the whole sold-out event was sponsored by his record label, Warner Records. Paul rounded up a cast of performers that included almost every major singing star of that generation: Bruce Springsteen, James Taylor, Billy Joel, Grand Funk, Dion, Lou Reed, and many others showed up and put on a spectacular show. There were a few star athletes, too, including the great Yankee captain Don Mattingly, then at the peak of his career and wildly popular.

Mattingly, like many of the performers, came out of the Garden's stage door close to where we had parked our mobile medical unit. But when he got to the unit, Don did something that has just stuck with me. Before climbing the stairs to get an inside look at the rolling clinic, he placed his hands on the outside of the unit, not saying anything. I was curious.

"Don, what was that about, I mean hands on the unit like that?"

"Well," said the slugger, "I was just appreciating how *real* this charity is. It's not theoretical or abstract. It's something very tangible. That means something to me."

That evening raised $500,000 for the Children's Health Fund. Generous superstars responded to Paul's call to action and ended up raising enough money to buy another mobile pediatric clinic and just about cover its first year's operating costs. We were about to double our impact, and I just hoped that Karen and the rest of our little team was ready for the ride of their lives.

I knew from the beginning of CHF that we needed to become a national initiative. Paul Simon said, "Take it easy. Let's just get it right in New York before we start thinking national." I understood the message, but didn't agree. The model in New York would be, from the outset, exportable anywhere. And we would establish certain principles that would apply going forward as the network grew: no compromise on the promise of excellent health care for every child, every day; utilization of advanced technology and mobile clinics to enhance services; affiliations with academic medical institutions; and a commitment to advocacy around access to care and the well-being of children.

To help move the national program and advocacy agenda forward, I hired Dennis Walto, a twenty-three-year-old, charming, highly organized former travel director for one-time presidential candidate Gary Hart. In 1990, Walto coordinated an extraordinary CHF caravan of vehicles that made a major road trip from New York City to Mississippi. The idea was to deliver a new mobile pediatric clinic to Clarksdale, accompanied by one of our New York City units, a fully wrapped tour bus, and some staff vehicles. We stopped in eight cities on the way down and in each location did lots of press, gave talks at medical facilities, and promoted the idea that all children needed access to health care.

Setting the stage for what would become a long-standing Redlener tradition of encouraging family volunteers, we also recruited David Redlener, then twenty-two years old, to join the caravan crew, serving as a trip logistic assistant to Walto. A second caravan in 1998 took a similar route and recruited my psychiatrist brother Neil as "trip videographer." Not to be left out, my youngest brother, Eric, a clinical psychologist, helped us design and implement mental health support programs for children who were traumatized by the terror attacks of 9/11.

Walto stayed with CHF for two years, helping to establish the CHF's national network of programs, then left for twenty-five years to run programs in Africa, the Middle East, and elsewhere, ultimately returning to become CHF's executive director in 2015.

In 1994, we brought on Dennis Johnson, one of my brother Eric's best friends and a smart, caring new colleague who would be instrumental in advancing the national network of mobile clinics for children. DJ eventually morphed into the person who kept CHF's advocacy agenda alive and thriving in Washington, DC.

Dennis Johnson and I shared one of the strangest experiences in the history of the Children's Health Fund. DJ and I were in Clarksdale, Mississippi, for a meeting in late 1998, and I had forgotten to bring a backup shirt for the dinner that was being organized for that evening. As we drove through the small town, we could see no store that would have what I needed. Then we spotted a forties-something, well-dressed white woman coming out of a dry cleaning store, and I said to Dennis, "Hey, slow down. I'll ask that lady if she knows where I can get a shirt."

"Hi. Excuse me, but we're wondering if there's someplace around here to buy a man's shirt?"

The lady walked over to the car, saw me in the passenger seat and Dennis, a particularly handsome African American man, driving, and said, very seriously, "If you mean a *white man's* shirt, you just won't find that around here. You'll need to go to Jackson or somewhere like that."

DJ and I cracked up laughing, and I ended up being the most underdressed dude at the dinner. Of course, it became a story that would be told and retold endlessly in the years ahead. Although it was funny to us, it was clearly a reminder that in terms of racism, or at least stereotypes and general insensitivity, America had a long way to go.

Carl Sagan and a New Children's Hospital in America's Poorest Urban Zip Code

One of the most gratifying, though entirely unexpected, outcomes of my work with Physicians for Social Responsibility (PSR) was a serendipitous meeting with the late astrophysicist Carl Sagan. In November 1981, university campus sit-ins were organized around the United States to call attention to the growing tension between the nuclear superpowers and the increasing possibility of a global nuclear war. Sagan, a brilliant, outspoken scientist and professor at Cornell University, was the star speaker and principal draw for the Cornell sit-in. I was invited to join Carl at the event, which attracted some fifteen hundred students and faculty; he focused on nuclear winter, and I on the impossibility of a medical response to nuclear war. The campus was totally energized. Carl, perhaps one of the most effective speakers I have ever heard, was powerful and compelling.

A number of people who had been at the event were invited to the astronomer's home for a reception and recap. The setting was stunning, with a wall of windows in the living room overlooking the cliffs of Ithaca. The conversation and wine were flowing, many of the guests chatting about the campus event and the existential threat posed by the arms race.

Because Karen and I would have had a long drive back to Utica from Ithaca, Carl and Ann Druyan, his wife, partner, and cowriter, invited us to spend the night at their home. When everyone else had gone, we spent a couple of hours talking with this uniquely gifted couple. The conversation was all over the place, sometimes serious, often hysterically funny—and personal. We got to know each other as we bonded over nukes and laughter and the follies of humanity.

What also struck me was the unabashed sensuality that permeated the space between and around Carl and Annie. Whether they were talking about their latest book, the relationship between religion and science, the joys and pains of academia, or our kids, the heat was on. Sitting there after midnight in the cliff house, operation central of this wildly in love and incredibly productive team of Carl and Annie, Inc., I was awed by the baritone-voiced, charismatic scientist laughing with his beautiful, brown-eyed writer partner. They did seem more or less aware of our presence and certainly made us feel welcome in the conversation, but I couldn't help feeling that Karen and I were clearly in their space.

Carl's voice, looks, and brilliance enthralled his students at Cornell—as well as the producers of late-night television, where he was a regular on nighttime talk shows. Ann was clearly a serious professional herself, an accomplished producer who co-wrote several books with Carl, as well as the screenplay for the star-studded hit movie *Contact*, a film that reflected the couple's passion and lifelong search for non-earthbound, nonhuman intelligent life in the universe.

No scientist, no public advocate, before or since Carl Sagan has had the combination of credibility and charisma he possessed and expressed so fluidly to any audience—millions watching him on TV, hundreds in classrooms, and some very lucky young people who had a chance to know Carl as a mentor. One of those mentees, a young, very bright kid from the Bronx, had written to Carl out of the blue saying that he, too, wanted to become an astronomer. "Come to Ithaca!" Carl responded. And that was how the now famous contemporary scientist and science advocate Neil de Grasse Tyson came to be friends with and mentee of Professor Sagan.

In the years that followed, Carl, Annie, Karen, and I became close friends, planning and plotting advocacy initiatives, always discussing politics and whatever else came up. One of Carl's most endearing habits was genuinely focusing on whoever was speaking. If he liked what he heard, he would pull a little notebook from his pocket and write down whatever was said that caught his interest. There might be something more gratifying than having a genius write down something you just said, but I don't know exactly what that would be.

A few years after meeting Carl and Ann, we let them know about our work with the Children's Health Fund, which would eventually become the nation's largest health care program utilizing mobile pediatric clinics to provide high-quality medical care for some of America's most disadvantaged children. They liked what they heard and eagerly accepted our offer to get involved. Ann served on CHF's board of directors, and Carl signed up as a member of the organization's advisory council.

Carl died of cancer in 1996 at the age of sixty-two, having left an indelible imprint on the world as an astute social observer, highly accomplished scientist, and humanist. Shortly before he died, I spoke with Carl, who was spending his last days at the Fred Hutchinson Cancer Center in Seattle. There was something he wanted to tell me.

"Irwin, I want you to know that I have gotten the best possible medical care that the world has to offer. Every possible option was explored for me, even if the outcome is now clear and the end is truly near. But I have been thinking how much attention and care I've received compared to how little so many children can depend on. So many kids don't have access even to the most basic care, no less the extraordinary attention I've gotten. Please keep working on fixing this terrible injustice."

For a moment I just couldn't speak. I was absorbing this powerful statement from an irreplaceable man, a giant, who was about to leave this world, who I once thought should be America's president, who influenced so many people, who wrote down clever things his friends said.

"Of course I will, Carl. Of course we all will."

The fact is that we were and are committed to a mission of providing high-quality health care to children. So, in a sense, all we needed to do to honor Carl's words was to keep providing the care as long as there was need. And, as far as we could see, out to and beyond the horizon, poverty and barriers to health care for vulnerable children weren't going to be eliminated any time soon. For all intents and purposes, or at least for the entirety of my professional career, inequities, disparities, and an absence of meaningful opportunities for poor people, especially poor minority children, were apparently here to stay. So we'd be here, too, bringing the care where it is needed most.

But I knew that wasn't what Carl was talking about when he exhorted me to keep fighting "this terrible injustice." He wasn't talking about giving vaccinations and checkups. That would be easy. That would be treading water. That would be my version of a Mother Teresa act—caring, unselfishly, for the marginalized and the hopeless, the ultimate humanitarian work defined by extreme kindness and caring to a degree that made her the symbol of self-lessness for the world. This was all good, representing a highly theological worldview, but it was not what Carl was asking—and not what I was intending to continue doing. Our mutual interest then, and mine still now, was upping the ante on the advocacy focus, even while continuing the clinical mission. We had to get the message fine-tuned, compelling, and clear. We needed to work upstream and at scale to change policies and priorities if we were actually to meet the challenges that seemed overwhelming and insoluble for so many children.

This was not about theology, or even sympathy and compassion. As a doctor, I had plenty of compassion—heartbreaking connections with children who were dying and suffering with health and economic adversities that were often beyond comprehension. I was in it for other reasons. How and when it started with me are complicated questions, but I was driven by a zero-tolerance attitude for injustice and disparities based on race, economic pressures, or ethnicity. My motivation for keeping the pressure on policy makers and the public to do the right thing by children has always been about fighting for civil rights, human rights, and equity, even if much of my career has been spent at the bedsides of children struggling for their lives, with families who couldn't care less about high-minded causes and social justice but just wanted me to be a doctor who knew what he was doing for the sole and focused purpose of saving their babies' lives. And that was very important to me.

No matter what else I was doing or standing for or advocating, I was confident in my medical skills. Knowing that I could take care of business with a very sick child was an essential aspect of my credibility as a competent professional, not just for the outside world, but for me on a highly personal basis. I never hesitated to exploit the fact that I was speaking as a doctor. That justified my self-righteousness and, perhaps, my authority at a Senate hearing on the health needs of homeless children or the need to reduce the possibility of nuclear war, or in writing a newspaper op-ed on children suffering in the aftermath of Hurricane Katrina.

In the early 1970s, I was confident that we would end child poverty in ten or fifteen years. I was in my late twenties then. By the time I got to my early seventies, it was clear that I was way off in my enthusiastic embrace of unfettered Kennedy-Johnson era optimism when it came to meeting massive social challenges. These fights are long haul and certainly not for the faint of heart. I was—and still am—easily seduced by serendipity, but I had to learn serious patience to survive in the real world of glacier-slow change, no matter how compelling the cause.

So what did happen after Carl Sagan and I spoke? Would his words resonate beyond his life? Certainly they have in the world at large. Untold numbers of young people were inspired to become scientists and proponents of a harmonious planet. Carl had a soaring hopefulness that transcended his clear awareness of how difficult it was to bring peace and enlightenment to the world.

Carl's influence was realized, too, in ways far more personal and directly connected to my own work. The first point of connection came in 1997, a year after Carl's death. I had been asked by the legendary president of Montefiore Medical Center, the late Dr. Spencer "Spike" Foreman, to take on leadership of an exciting new project. The idea was to build the first-ever children's hospital in the Bronx, one of New York City's "outer boroughs" and home to the poorest urban zip codes in the United States. Some 400,000 children were among the Bronx's population, the majority in families living well below the poverty line. Access to care, especially advanced subspecialty care, had long been a challenge for these children, and a new hospital dedicated to them and the borough would be a groundbreaking advance for the community.

Taking this on would not be easy. I would be leading a group of hospital insiders who were longtime fixtures at Montefiore. For the most part, these people were highly competent and dedicated to the institution's mission of community service. Many of them outranked me in the hospital's hierarchy.

"Why me?" I asked Spike in a long one-on-one conversation we had about the new hospital's leadership.

"I trust you. I trust the others, too, of course," he responded, "but I trust you to build something unique and beautiful, a place for children's health care that goes beyond the routine cookie-cutter design."

"The other point, Irwin, is that this effort will cost well over $100 million, and I will need your help in raising that money." He smiled at that—and so did I. We clearly understood each other.

Two things followed from that conversation. The first was that I reached out to one of the most creative and successful designers of public and commercial buildings in the United States, David Rockwell. David loved the idea of participating in this project, and his entire creative staff was made available to work with the Montefiore team. The second outcome was an idea I had a few months after accepting Foreman's offer. It literally occurred to me when I was drifting off to sleep one night in early 1997, before any design commitments had been made or even discussed. This new hospital should be all about Carl Sagan's wishes for planetary peace, the search for truth, and promoting a sense of hopefulness and yearning for equity in a tough and challenging world.

The next day, I called Carl's widow and laid out the concept.

"Ann, here's what I'm imagining for this new hospital that is being built for the children of the Bronx. Yes, it will be a place of healing, primarily, of course. It will have every modern medical capacity that a new children's hospital should. It will be built around the needs and comfort of the children—and their families. This means large single rooms that accommodate parents staying with their children for the duration of their hospitalization. We call that 'family-centered care.' "

"Sounds good. I'm sure it will be beautiful and a great place for care."

"Well, there's more," I said. "The theme of the whole hospital—what it does, how it looks, and the messages it delivers—will be designed around the issues that Carl stood for. This could be the Children's Hospital at Montefiore *and* something we'd call the Carl Sagan Discovery Center."

"I love the idea. Tell me more."

I went on to lay out more exactly what I had in mind. The new hospital would be built to promote, overtly and otherwise, the idea of learning and discovery, much of it built around, but not limited to, health sciences. We would work with the design consultants, David Rockwell's group, to make every floor, every room, and all the common spaces opportunities for children and youth to be inspired by science, to learn, and to think that their own futures had extraordinary possibilities they might have never considered before.

This new children's hospital would be like no other—a place of great medical care and comfortable healing, but also a place of inspiration.

I recruited my longtime information technology guru, Jeb Weisman, to immerse himself in the design process. It was Jeb who came up with conceptual and implementation strategies for bedside access to flat screen monitors, allowing children and families to avail themselves of many opportunities not only to learn about the conditions they had but also to explore the world as they were recovering. All of this was extremely innovative in the mid-1990s. Jeb hired young college students from the neighborhood to act as doyens, or explainers, and trained them to guide and teach the younger patients. The whole program was a rousing success.

Rockwell's group commissioned extraordinary art installations and placed them throughout the new hospital. A giant Foucault perpetual pendulum, designed and built by the famed sculpture Tom Otterness, was set in the multilevel atrium. An enormous biosphere was in the main lobby, with smaller pieces, art boxes, and interactive displays placed throughout.

At the opening of the new hospital in 2001, just weeks after the 9/11 terror attacks, with the piles of rubble that had once been the majestic World Trade Center still smoldering, I sat behind the podium up in the northwest Bronx waiting to speak, overwhelmed by the searing tragedy of that nightmare in downtown Manhattan but so deeply proud of the work of art and citadel of health care for children that the hospital team had made real. This tribute to the well-being of vulnerable children, at the same time presenting something of a pathway for them to envision a future of possibility, seemed to me an antidote to the evil of 9/11.

What made it even more poignant for me was that it fulfilled a promise to Sagan. He wanted us to keep working the mission, to make the Earth a place of promise and fulfillment, and to put the health care available to a child in the Bronx on the same level of excellence he had received as a famous world leader in one of the nation's most prestigious hospitals. The children's hospital turned out to be a huge success, deeply appreciated by the community and the medical staff. By 2015, Montefiore's dynamic new CEO, Steve Safyer, was already thinking about raising funds to double the size of Children's Hospital.

"Yes, Carl," I thought, "I remember, and we're on our way."

Sagan's influence persisted in some very unusual ways and continued to reinforce my basic philosophy that serendipity was irresistible as long as it didn't distract from ongoing projects that must continue. Two years into the children's hospital project, and two years before the ribbon cutting, another Sagan-related opportunity came about in the strangest of ways.

Dinner with Fidel

It seems that the long-standing dictator-president of Cuba, Fidel Castro, was an avid reader of all genres, from deep philosophical works to historical analysis and science. He fancied himself a literary critic, a philosopher-ruler, an international figure of standing and import, an observer of the world and all its foibles. In particular, he was a serious fan of Carl Sagan, having read most of his work. Castro had always wanted to meet Sagan in person but never made arrangements to do so prior to Carl's untimely demise.

Reportedly frustrated by this failure to meet Carl, Fidel came up with an alternative. In 1999, three years after Sagan's death, Fidel reached out to his old friend Joan Campbell, then head of the National Council of Churches, to help convey an invitation to Ann Druyan, Carl's widow. In lieu of meeting with Sagan himself, the Cuban leader would settle for Annie.

Ann was intrigued and said she would go, but only if she could bring along her children and a few friends. The Cubans agreed. Ann immediately called me, described the opportunity, and asked if Karen and I would like to join her. "Yes!" was my immediate response.

There wasn't a chance I wouldn't accept. This was an irresistible opportunity to visit the mysterious island nation, a declared enemy of the United States for more than half a century, sitting just ninety miles off the Florida coast. And we would be official guests of Fidel Castro himself! Extraordinary.

But there was more. Cuba had a global reputation for a highly effective, distributive health care system, meaning widespread accessible community health care throughout the country and universal preventive care, including extremely high rates of vaccinated children. In addition, medical education in Cuba had a well-deserved reputation for academic rigor, producing well-trained doctors who graduated from medical school with a purposeful sense of community service. And by design, the production of doctors from Cuba's medical schools far exceeded the nation's own needs. Castro's idea was to create a pipeline of doctors who could serve around the world in countries where health challenges were extreme but physicians and other health care providers were in extremely short supply.

Needless to say, beyond the humanitarian rhetoric rationalizing these policies, the political ramifications of this global health assistance outreach, especially in South America and Africa, were a powerful motivator. In fact, this idea of influencing hearts and minds through strategic humanitarian intervention has increasingly been deployed by other nations, including the United States. When serving as U.S. secretary of state, Hillary Clinton promoted the idea of "global health diplomacy." In a sense, this approach can be understood as a nonmilitary pathway to extending a nation's interests and influence globally.

In addition to meeting long-term health care access objectives, providing significant disaster relief has the same effect. Like the United States, Japan, France, Israel, and many other countries, Cuba is almost always among the first in line to provide medical assistance in the face of large-scale disasters. In this arena, they are consistently seen as highly competent and collaborative.

It's even more impressive to understand that Cuba's national system of ubiquitous access to health care and its extensive international efforts to support health care capacity in economically struggling regions across the globe have been accomplished in spite of extreme and chronic national economic stress and shortages of material goods, including certain medical supplies, in Cuba itself. Clearly, the decades-long U.S.-imposed embargo contributed to Cuba's economic morass, particularly after the collapse of the former Soviet Union, once a major contributor to Cuba's economy. During the heyday of the USSR, Cuba, as another of its "client states," benefited greatly. Yet, despite these pressures, not only has Cuba maintained its global reputation as an exporter of quality health care, it has also developed a world-class medical research capacity, including breakthroughs in vaccine production and state-of-the-art innovations in the treatment of cancer.

So yes, I was intrigued by the whole idea of visiting Cuba. Above all, I was interested in seeing for myself what this mysterious country and its notorious dictator had created in terms of its unique health, public health, and medical research systems that, in many ways, have been so remarkably effective. In particular, I wanted to see how Cuba's advanced public health system affected the health, and especially the well-being, of children.

Needless to say, Karen and I enthusiastically let Ann know that we would be thrilled to join her on the trip to Cuba, but we had two caveats: we wanted to bring our friends Bobby and Carol Tannenhauser, and most important, I wanted assurances that we'd have an opportunity to see Cuba's health care system in action.

Annie agreed to our proposal to bring Carol and Bobby, and the Cubans agreed to the terms and conditions related to what we wanted to see. Fidel, they explained, was so determined to have an in-person meeting with Sagan's widow that he would comply with all requests. And that's how it came to be that for a week in early February of 1999, a small group of Ann Druyan's intrepid friends and family members ended up on an entirely unique field trip to Cuba, sanctioned because of the connection to the U.S. Council of Churches but motivated by a chance to witness, to observe firsthand, the massive intellectual curiosity, insatiable ego, and unabashed hubris of the world's longest serving, former revolutionary, stalwart communist national leader/dictator.

It all came off as we hoped it would. We were treated like VIPs, "escorted"—or closely watched—by Castro's minders, but we talked to many everyday Cubans; ate in Havana's inner-city restaurants; visited a synagogue, where they told us of Fidel's many long visits to spend time with the elders discussing Hebraic theology; toured the main children's hospital, where we spoke with heart surgeons who asked me to send them some equipment they needed; drove to an outlying rural health center; visited with scientists in a premier medical research center; and talked in hushed voices with CIA operatives in the so-called United States Interests Section of the Embassy of Switzerland in Havana, Cuba.

Then, on Thursday, we got "the call." El Presidente invited the Druyan party to join him for dinner at the presidential palace. For nearly seven hours, the nine travelers chatted with Fidel in the anteroom and then were seated with him and his translator at the long wooden table in the grand dining room—all because of Castro's unrequited admiration for Carl Sagan, the philosopher-humanist-scientist whom he dreamed of meeting but never did.

On the evening of the dinner, members of Castro's staff drove us to the presidential palace, where we waited for thirty minutes before being invited into the anteroom for cocktails, not expecting to see Fidel before dinner. Then, to our surprise and with little fanfare, he strode into the room and immediately engaged us all in conversation. The leader was beyond charming, dressed in green combat fatigues, including his field hat, looking every bit the part of a military officer heading back to his troops.

Clearly, Castro was most interested in speaking with Annie. The repartee between them was fascinating, ranging from discussions of Carl's work to Greek philosophers and George Soros's latest book. He repeatedly challenged Ann on almost every subject, including what Soros stood for and what he was trying to say in his book. But Ann was more than his equal, besides which she and Carl knew Soros personally. She told Fidel that "George Soros got his ideas from Karl Popper," followed by a long mini-lecture covering a wide range of related issues.

Our friend, journalist Carol Tannenhauser, who wrote brilliantly about this trip and our dinner with President Castro, described it this way: "Fidel stopped talking and turned to look at her [Annie], surprise, scrutiny and interest in his eyes. He seemed to consider in that moment that he might just have met a mind that was a match for his own." After Ann delivered a brilliant discourse on Karl Popper, Carl Sagan, and a good bit about ancient philosophers, Carol went on, "Fidel's eyes lit up. There were intellectuals in the house. It was time for dinner."[6]

And what a dinner it was—just our little group, Fidel and his translator extraordinaire, a petite middle-aged woman who had worked with him for nearly thirty years. The translation from Spanish to English was rendered almost simultaneously with Castro's own words, to the point that we quickly lost track of the fact that there was even a translator present.

Fidel talked almost incessantly during the dinner, which lasted until nearly 4:00 a.m. He talked about the building of Cuba and the nation's many accomplishments in science, and, to our great surprise, he was happy to show off his substantial fluency when it came to American politics, including knowing a good bit about the Electoral College system and the likely candidates for the 2000 U.S. presidential elections that were still some nine months in the future.

About three hours into the dinner, Castro abruptly turned to me. "So, what exactly do you do, Dr. Redlener?" he asked, his hands clasped on the table in front of him.

"Well, right now, I'm working on planning and building the first-ever children's hospital in an area of New York City called the Bronx," I answered.

"I know of it," Fidel said. "It is a place of great poverty."

"That's right. In fact, it is the poorest urban community in America. Many children have very limited access to medical care, and there has never been a designated children's hospital in that borough before, even though it is home to some 400,000 children."

"You're saying, many of those children do not have medical care?" Fidel asked.

"Nearly 20 million children in America do not have access to the kind of timely, comprehensive care they need," I replied.

"I am truly sorry to hear that," he said. "But I won't talk about those statistics you cited. I wouldn't want to get you in trouble! By the way," he joked, "I would be happy to send some of our wonderful doctors to help you in the Bronx."

I cringed. Was Fidel Castro mocking me?

"How many beds will you have in your new hospital?" the president asked.

"We're planning on 120 to start with, leaving room for growth when the time comes."

"How many pediatric ICU beds are you planning on putting in?" Fidel asked.

"Right now, it looks like about twenty," I said.

"Twenty?" Fidel repeated. "That's too many for the population, not to mention the overall size of the hospital."

What was going on here? I couldn't believe I was sitting there engaged in a conversation with Fidel Castro about the details of hospital planning in New York City!

"Actually, Mr. President," I said, "if we do go for the twenty, between six and eight will be 'step-down' beds for children recovering from intensive care or just not sick enough for the ICU management protocols." Take that!

Fidel stroked his beard. "Ah! I understand. Makes sense. . . ."

"One more point, Mr. President. The new hospital will be dedicated to Carl Sagan. We're creating a real showcase of discovery and learning for children who must be confined to the hospital," I added.

He nodded to me but turned to Karen, "Are you working on the hospital, too?"

"No," she replied. "I'm one of the leaders of a national network of clinics and mobile units that bring health care to some of America's most disadvantaged communities. We've been at it for about twelve years now. And the new Sagan hospital will back our mobile program for children who need more advanced medical care."

"Very good," Fidel said, admiringly. "I hope you will get a chance to see some of our clinics before you leave. You know, it's not only the medical follow-up that's important. You should follow those children back into their communities and see if what was inspired by the Sagan hospital can be carried into their future educations."

"That's a very good idea," Karen said.

Fidel nodded and smiled, then turned back to me. "How are you paying for your hospital?"

"We're raising about $120 million from individuals and some from the government."

"I see," Fidel said. "Well, I suggest that you collect the money— not just pledges—soon. The U.S. economy is fragile, and the stock market is showing great instability. If you don't get the money now, you might not be able to collect on some of the promises later."

Through it all, I was formulating a question and didn't want to leave without asking it.

"Mr. President," I blurt out, "to be sure, I am well aware of the extraordinary advances Cuba has made in its ability to ensure that no citizen goes without access to health care. I also know your doctors are highly trained and capable, and the whole world is well aware of how you have dispatched Cuban medical teams to many countries in need, where doctors are in short supply."

"The thing is," I said, "there have been many claims made about disparities between what average Cuban citizens, those struggling economically, receive from Cuba's health care system and the quality of care available to senior government and military officials and so-called health tourists. What can you say about that?"

Fidel shrugged and glanced toward the ceiling, shaking his head, seeming slightly bemused. Then he spoke with particular care and emphasis.

"I can say with complete assurance that it is not true," he said. "Every Cuban citizen has access to whatever medical care he or she needs. It is true that we have shortages everywhere in the system, especially of certain medicines and medical supplies and parts for advanced equipment. That is where the American embargo has been most painful for me."

There would be no way to prove my assertion—or his response—one way or the other in the short time we had in Cuba. I had to leave it as I had started—an assertion likely to be true, but maybe not.

No matter what, we had a unique experience and an opportunity to spend quality time with one of history's most complex figures, a leftist dictator at our front door, a revolutionary hero who four decades earlier had defeated a right-wing dictator, Fulgencio Batista, creating a social and political experiment that remains a work in progress.

If it weren't for a moment of outright serendipity, a chance opportunity to share a stage nearly twenty years earlier with Carl Sagan, one of America's most influential voices on the danger of nuclear war, we would not have found ourselves at the dinner table with a man who was a central figure in the Cuban Missile Crisis, a leader who would eventually go to his grave as much of an enigma as he was to us that cool February night on the outskirts of Havana.

Fidel Castro died of natural causes at age ninety on November 25, 2016. I couldn't help remembering how much the lifelong revolutionary, brilliant innovator, intolerant, often cruel, totalitarian leader, and proud Cuban patriot was obsessed with dying before the CIA could kill him. He got his wish. He lived for nearly two years after President Barack Obama took steps to begin normalizing the relationship between the United States and the island nation that Fidel had nurtured and controlled through the second half of the twentieth century.

As for Carl Sagan, through the years that I knew him, when he was a living inspiration and a vibrant social force, his influence on me was unbounded, and—to an extent that still surprises me—it remains true so many years after his death. I know this because I still talk with students and colleagues about Sagan's deep concern about the environmental impact of nuclear conflict, because I often reread his pale blue dot essay on the need for us to remain humble in the face of the inestimable vastness of the universe, and because of how very often I recall his deathbed words about inequities suffered by the world's vulnerable children. Carl Sagan indeed lives on, for me and who knows how many others around the world.

Elian Gonzalez: Political Child Abuse and an International Uproar

It was a particularly busy afternoon in late March 2000 when my assistant let me know that I had a call from the Immigration and Naturalization Service (INS) commissioner. I couldn't imagine why she'd be calling me, but my curiosity was piqued.

"Dr. Redlener, I'm Doris Meissner of the INS, and we could use your help. My boss, Attorney General Janet Reno, and I are hoping you'll be able to help us in the matter of Elian Gonzalez. Are you familiar with the situation?"

How could I not be? Elian's story was in the news every day and had been since the six-year-old had survived the capsizing of a small boat with emigrants attempting to escape Cuba, headed for South Florida. His mother and eight others had died when the small boat took on water during a major storm surge. Initially young Elian was turned over to distant relatives in Miami who, with the intense support of the Cuban American community, decided to make the custody—and citizenship—of the six-year-old the centerpiece of a highly publicized ideological battle between vehemently anti-Castro hard-right activists and almost everyone else. Elian's father, Juan Miguel Gonzalez Quintana, had come to Washington, DC, hoping to take his son back home to Havana; Elian's Miami family and their supporters, on the other hand, were doing everything they could to secure U.S. citizenship for the child and block his return to Cuba.

Unfortunately for Elian, he had become a symbol of this enormous uproar. The Miami "family" kept him confined to their small Miami home, occasionally parading him on someone's shoulders at all hours of the day and night. They seemed intent on refighting their grievances with Castro through the plight and fate of this boy.

Commissioner Meissner and the attorney general wanted my help in assembling a small group of mental health experts to interview Elian's father, just to confirm that he was fit to have custody of the boy. The Miami family's all-out effort to secure a legal or legislative hold on Elian was failing. The U.S. government could not justify any reason to keep him from returning to Cuba, so reaching out to me was a way to inoculate federal officials against potential allegations that Juan was incapable of raising his own son.

I agreed to help. My first step was to ask Lourdes Rigal-Lynch, a very capable child psychologist who worked for us at the Children's Health Fund, to help identify a team of well-reputed bilingual experts to interview Juan Miguel and participate in a report for the attorney general stating that Elian's father was or was not capable of parenting. The group of evaluators, Drs. Ian Camino of Columbia University, Paulina Kernberg, and Dr. Luis Polo of

Albert Einstein College of Medicine met with Juan Miguel and concurred that he was, indeed, a fit parent.

Meanwhile, the demands that Elian be forbidden to return to Cuba were getting increasingly out of control and angry, with large, sign-carrying crowds parading in front of the Miami family's house. On April 14, 2000, the Miami relatives released a most peculiar video purported to be a "spontaneous statement" by Elian stating that he didn't want to go back to Cuba. Off-camera voices were heard coaching him on what to say.

A few days later, the Saturday following release of the video, Karen and I were at a restaurant with our friends Bobby and Carol Tannenhauser. I was talking about the Elian situation and this latest videotape.

"You know, I am really concerned about this kid and the impact all of this public drama is going to have on him," I said to the three of them. "I don't even think he's going to school. He's being totally exploited to make a political point. The fact is that this child is being psychologically abused. It's more than apparent just from what we're seeing on the news."

"So what would you do if this wasn't the strange, high-profile situation that it has become?" Bobby responded.

"Well, I would certainly be ready to call Child Protective Services and let them make a decision about removing that child from that crazy environment."

"OK. That's my point," Bobby responded. "Maybe you should 'call it in' and let the attorney general know what you're thinking."

On the way home, Karen and I talked about how to handle the possibility of formally characterizing what was happening with Elian as psychological abuse. The situation was at a stalemate. Reno and Meissner wanted the child turned over to the father and allowed to return to Cuba. The Miami family, increasingly strident, were holding fast to their position and refusing to release Elian to authorities. No definitive court decision was in sight. By the time we got home, I knew what I needed to do.

The next day, Sunday, I drafted a letter outlining my concerns and faxed it to the attorney general late that evening.

The letter said in part:

Elian Gonzalez is now in a state of imminent danger to his physical and emotional well-being in a home that I consider to be psychologically abusive. In a less politically charged environment . . . appropriate child welfare workers and other public officials would have already been called upon to evaluate the safety of the current environment, and, in my view, would have [already] removed Elian. . . .

Therefore, in my professional judgement, the United States government . . . should:

1. *Immediately remove Elian Gonzalez from the custody of Lazaro Gonzalez. . . .*
2. *Return Elian to the custody of his biologic father . . . as quickly as possible. Our country has no reason and no right to continue this unconscionable refutation of a parent's moral right to be with his child.*

Within hours, the attorney general released the letter to the press, setting off a firestorm of angry reaction and counterreaction. I did dozens of interviews with print journalists and morning network TV reporters. The right-wing press and commentators were merciless, accusing me of making a diagnosis without examining the child (totally unnecessary in this case). I was called a communist and a fraud and was getting threatening messages at home and at the office, to the point that I was assigned U.S. Marshal protection, including agents stationed outside my home.

This was an intense and unsettling experience, but I never regretted speaking out. I knew what I saw, and I knew that Elian needed to be with his father, even if it meant a return to Cuba. And I was struck by the hypocrisy of the right-wing Cuban

American "resistors." These were the people who always fought for the supremacy of the family, for the rights of parents to make their own decisions about how to manage and raise their own children. Now, to make an unwinnable ideological point and use a six-year-old's tragedy as an exploitable new opportunity to take on Fidel Castro, principles of family values and a nonintervening government were set aside.

For me, Castro was an iconoclastic dictator and a very mixed bag for the Cuban people. But Juan Miguel and Elian were still father and son and, for that reason alone, deserved to be reunited and free to go.

There was yet one more, very odd piece of this story. I had been working hard as a volunteer and surrogate speaker for Al Gore's 2000 presidential campaign and, in that role, was in regular contact with campaign officials, and occasionally Gore himself. When the Elian case was heating up, I let the team know that I was going to be "out there" very publicly in support of returning Elian to his father's custody. I also made the point that I thought this would be a good issue for Mr. Gore to speak out on. It was apparent to most voters, I thought, that father and son should be reunited. In spite of the volume of protest from the Cuban American community, most Floridians would agree with reunification.

That was the last communication I had with Gore's campaign, on any level. I was cut off and never again acknowledged as representing the candidate in any forum. The problem was that Gore was flip-flopping—initially favoring the effort to keep Elian in the United States, then changing his mind and supporting Janet Reno's position of extracting the boy from the clutches of the Miami family who claimed him.

Gore's vacillation and refusal to articulate what he likely believed may have had a defining impact on the outcome of the 2000 presidential election. It all hung on the bizarre vote counting in one of the most important swing states of that election cycle. The former vice president gambled on the belief that voters would turn against him if he pushed for reunification. That turned out to be a bad and unprincipled wager that brought George W. Bush to the White House. In a *New York Times* article on the matter published on March 29, 2000, reporter Katharine Q. Seelye's lede was "Could Vice President Al Gore's fate be tied to that of a 6-year-old boy from Cuba?"

I'm afraid that's precisely what happened.

Perhaps the most important takeaway from this entire incident with Elian was an intense national focus on the welfare of children. Was Elian being abused and exploited? I strongly believed so. Should he have been immediately returned to his father's custody? Of course. When angry partisans demanded that Elian remain in the United States because they so despised Cuba and Fidel Castro, my colleagues and I saw that as subordinating the well-being of a little boy to a political and ideological agenda. Getting that child back home with his father became a moral and ethical fight we weren't about to lose.

Fleeing to Disasters

In 1975, I was given a chance to take a group of University of Miami medical students to a remote rural community in Honduras, one of the poorest countries in the Western Hemisphere. The idea was to mentor the students in an elective experience where they would learn about how rural poverty, subsistence living, food and water insecurity, and a very poor medical system conspired to make life unspeakably difficult for children and families. There was much to learn in Santa Rosa de Copan—for the students and for me, too. We saw profound poverty in the capital and more of the same in the surrounding farming villages. We made rounds in the pediatric wards of the town's only hospital, horrified by the lack of supplies and trained personnel and by seeing two, sometimes three, very sick babies lying on a bare mattress in a single crib.

During and after rounds, we spent a great deal of time discussing vitamin deficiencies, diarrheal disease from contaminated water, and exotic infections that brought these children to the hospital. Almost every day at least one child would die in that forlorn hospital, while we—and the regular hospital staff—were essentially powerless to provide more than the most basic medical care.

But the essential lessons here were not about how to provide better acute care, though it was impossible not to talk about these issues every day on hospital rounds. What mattered from a teaching perspective—and what constantly reminded me of the challenges I faced in Lee County, Arkansas—was learning to understand the preconditions, the social determinants of health that created the medical crises playing out on the pediatric wards of the hospital. In this setting, it was nearly impossible to successfully manage the acute medical needs of any individual child. Nutritional recovery, vitamin replacement therapy, and antibiotics were all indicated, but by the time we saw those children in the hospital, they were in extremis. It was too late to save them—even if the medicines and supplements had been available, which they weren't.

We were looking at individual children who needed but couldn't get appropriate medical care—but what was really needed were strategies designed to understand and manage the upstream conditions that led to the catastrophic cases we saw in the hospital. Good doctors and medical teams were always necessary, but it would take experts in economic development and public health to address the big-picture challenges behind the tragedies that played out on the squalid pediatric wards there in Santa Rosa.

It was there that a very angry young soldier pointed his assault rifle at me, demanding that I leave "his hospital." At the time, it didn't feel to me that this showdown would necessarily end well. One of the nurses calmed the teenager down and escorted him back to his unit, which happened to be based at the hospital. There wasn't another episode like that while we were there, but it left a serious impression on the students—and me. Oddly enough, we never found out what the boy soldier was so angry about, but, fortunately, we never saw him again.

A year later, a 7.5 Richter earthquake rocked a rural mountainous region in Guatemala, some hundred miles from the capital, Guatemala City. Mass fatalities and serious injuries, destroyed villages, and appeals for assistance were being reported by the news media, often punctuated by heart-stopping videos of the wreckage. The disaster was getting the world's attention—and I couldn't help wondering if there was something I could or should do to help. I turned to a colleague on the medical school faculty, David Taplin, a researcher in the department of dermatology. Taplin had vast experience working in remote regions, both with the U.S. Army and as a volunteer in many disaster relief efforts.

"David, the situation in Guatemala is horrendous. Can we do something?" I asked.

"Probably. What do you have in mind?"

"If I can identify a few medical volunteers, can you handle the logistics to get us down there and make sure we're appropriately connected to authorities in charge?"

"Sure," he said with characteristic confidence.

It turned out that I found enough doctors, nurses, and med students to staff two teams, each fully equipped with what was needed to function with minimal support from local authorities. Within forty-eight hours, Professor Taplin had gotten everything organized, and we were on our way. He took charge of one team, I the other.

Once on the ground, we connected with both Guatemalan and U.S. military units who were already providing urgent medical assistance.

The scene was pure chaos. Rescue teams were coming in from around the world, and very little of the incoming personnel management and resources were centrally coordinated. Two airport hangars were literally filled with piles of useless donations, from stockings and battery-operated toys to lipstick and outdated medication samples. None of it was sorted in any way, and nobody had any idea of what should be done with any of these essentially useless, though perhaps well-meaning, donations.

Our task was to get to the hard-hit areas, set up makeshift medical facilities, and get to work trying to help as many of the disaster victims as we could. Transportation arrangements for us, at least, were less problematic than I had expected. Both U.S. and Guatemalan helicopter crews seemed willing to take us to the disaster zones. We stayed in Guatemala City, left for the mountain villages early in the morning and returned at sundown, staying overnight in the cheapest hotel we could find.

Villagers were receptive and grateful—and we treated hundreds of survivors. A serious continuing challenge was a constant state of seismic instability. Literally thousands of aftershocks were recorded, and the villagers were terrified. We were, too, but tried hard not to show how anxious we were, focusing as much as we could on getting our medical facilities set up and functioning.

The realities were sobering. We saw countless victims with serious injuries, many needing transport to the capital for advanced medical and surgical treatment. But what took the biggest emotional toll on our teams were the stories related by villagers who had lost loved ones, especially children who had perished and many others still not accounted for.

The lessons were there for the taking. Guatemala was not prepared for a disaster of this scale. Buildings made of unreinforced adobe in a known seismic zone became death traps when the earthquake struck. Critical supplies were difficult to come by, and the mountains of useless materials in the airport hangars at the capital were a serious management problem. From our perspective, a major problem was a serious lack of coordination among national agencies, international assistance, and nongovernmental organizations.

We returned to Miami exhausted and dismayed. That said, I would not soon forget what we had seen. Insights were gained the hard way about what to do—and especially what *not* to do—in preparing for and responding to a major disaster. Both interesting and disturbing was a detailed report by the U.S. comptroller general's office to the Congress on relief efforts in response to the 1976 earthquake. The problems described in the report were significant, from poor coordination of agencies to unmet communications challenges, all findings that were important and essential to learn from. But most concerning is the fact that many of the problems identified decades ago remain still unresolved, reappearing over and over again in other major disasters across the globe, including the 2004 Indonesian tsunami, Hurricane Katrina on the U.S. Gulf Coast in 2005, and the 2010 earthquake in Haiti.

The work of disaster preparedness and response, while frustrating and difficult in so many ways, was nonetheless exhilarating and deeply rewarding. What was going on? How did my desire to respond to major disasters relate to my primary job at the time—directing a pediatric intensive care unit in Miami some thousand miles northeast of Guatemala City?

Doctors attracted to emergency medicine, intensive care, or trauma surgery are among those professionals who seek and are sustained by being on the front lines of situations where lives are literally and immediately at stake. Perhaps there's an internally rewarding hormonal cocktail of adrenaline and endorphins at play here. Maybe, too, there is an overdose of hubris and an experience-based, acquired sense of confidence, merited or not, that comes from being a doctor whose actions can make a difference between life and death. For the right personality, this kind of medical practice is addictive and self-reinforcing when there's success, when a life has been saved. But if the outcome is not good, there is a tendency to explain what happened in ways that take the onus off oneself. "He was too far gone when he got here"; "They screwed up her care in the other hospital"; "We did everything we could."

Professionals who rush toward the big disasters are sometimes called brave. They want to save lives, and they put themselves in harm's way to help others. Many are true heroes, and most are true humanitarians. But they can also be "crisis addicts," much as ICU and ER doctors, SWAT teams, firefighters, and special forces are. This is not meant to disparage. Society is extremely lucky to have a lot of men and women who live for the adventure. We should celebrate the "can-dos" and "will-dos" who walk among us!

If this kind of attraction to hard-core emergencies is an affliction, I think that somewhere along the way, in the chronic disasters of southeast Arkansas and rural Honduras, through drought and famine in sub-Saharan Africa, and working in the aftermath of the big earthquake in Guatemala, I picked up a touch of that particular crisis virus. Disaster response clearly appealed to me, then and now.

What I struggled with, though, was that I was still very much drawn to addressing the challenges of socially vulnerable children who must cope with chronic adversities powerful enough to shut down opportunity pathways. Poor health and reduced access to health care, undernutrition, and bad schools—the well-known effects of poverty—can sabotage a child's life chances. But unlike natural disasters or pandemics that, while dangerous and life-threatening, are most often unpredictable and unavoidable, poverty and its consequences can be definitively addressed and overcome. In fact, confronting the precursors of social, economic, and political crises, as slow motion disasters for children and families, is as compelling to me as caring for a child in an ICU or responding to a major natural disaster.

All of these are emergencies that require immediate action, all are complex events that involve overlapping challenges. For instance, poor children are especially vulnerable in major disasters. A major storm with flooding threatens an entire community. But families with limited resources are far more at risk than non-poor, better-resourced families.

214

Child poverty has been a problem in America for generations, and at this point it may seem to be a nearly insoluble, fixed social condition. I don't buy that assumption. For me, finding solutions and opening up opportunities for all children to fulfill their potential and realize their aspirations is a realistic goal and, furthermore, a matter of great urgency. In fact, it is the call to urgent action that is the common ground shared by the desire to break the cycle of child poverty, to care for a child who needs intensive medical care, or to respond to a disaster when vulnerable children are at risk.

When category 5 Hurricane Andrew struck South Florida in 1992, I deployed one of CHF's New York mobile clinics and a medical team led by one of our most capable physicians, Dr. Alan Shapiro. Working with Paul Simon's friend, former chairman of the Joint Chiefs of Staff Colin Powell, we were in the thick of the response and recovery efforts. Responding to a major disaster by focusing on the care and well-being of the most vulnerable children in the affected communities accommodates the need to respond to a crisis and, at the same time, do whatever it takes to protect children at risk.

And then there was 9/11. A case could be made that no sentient person on the planet was unaffected by the highly organized terror attacks against the United States. Like ripples and waves, from the inner circles of death and destruction in New York, Washington, DC, and Shanksville, Pennsylvania, to the families and friends of the killed and injured, to the neighborhoods close to, but not directly hit by, the hijacked planes, the trauma was immediate and persistent. Many people referred to the World Trade Center and the Pentagon as "ground zero." Those were the physical targets. But there was also a virtual ground zero, in that the psychological and societal impact extended well beyond the physical destruction in and around the immediate vicinity of the smoldering piles. Sadly, the widespread emotional trauma made the complex attack of September 11, 2001, the perfect terror event.

Within twenty-four hours of the jetliners' hitting the World Trade Center towers, we deployed two mobile medical units to assist in the triage services set up just blocks from the burning pile. These triage teams saw far fewer patients than had been anticipated; people had either perished or survived with relatively minimal immediate medical needs. However, when the acute crisis was over, many children in New York remained deeply traumatized and emotionally unsettled by the understandably incessant coverage of the 9/11 attacks and their aftermath. Because mental health services and support for children were so limited in New York City, especially in low-income neighborhoods, Karen set up a mobile pediatric mental health evaluation and treatment program funded by the Red Cross, the Robin Hood Foundation, and others. Paula Madrid, a terrific young psychologist working under the supervision of my psychologist brother, Eric, was recruited to develop and run the program.

After responding to Hurricane Andrew in 1992 and in the aftermath of the 9/11 terrorism, CHF leadership had a lot to think about, ultimately deciding to add another explicit element to our organizational mission: a commitment to respond to public health crises when vulnerable children were at risk. Beyond that, the relationships among disaster risk, resiliency, and vulnerable children were becoming increasingly intriguing to me and would soon influence my next career move.

In a strange timing juxtaposition, the 9/11 attacks preceded by just a few weeks the opening of the new children's hospital in the Bronx. In took an enormous institution-wide team to get the first-ever children's hospital in that borough designed and built, but I had the lead design responsibility for the new facility and had been designated its president. That's really why I was invited to a special briefing on September 25 designed to update health system representatives from every hospital in the region regarding the status of the recovery, plans to safeguard against other threats, and an assessment of needs in medical systems and the community at large.

For several hours, representatives from key federal, state, and local agencies presented perspectives and explanations for what was going to happen going forward. Finally, it was time for Q & A. I was sitting in the back of the room next to a close and long-time colleague, Alan Rosenfield, the late, highly respected dean of Columbia's Mailman School of Public Health. We had been kibitzing throughout the presentations.

At one point Alan put his hand on my knee, turned to me, and said, "Irwin, I am telling you this right now, I don't believe we are remotely prepared for terrorism, or any other kind of major disaster. We barely think about such things at the School, but we've got to get a handle on this. Every disaster is a threat to people, especially those who are already vulnerable. I've seen this all over the world."

"I agree—and you need to fix that."

So when we were finally invited to ask questions, my hand was in the air—and I was called on first.

"Thank you for the opportunity to ask a question; and mine is simple. What preparations have been made or are being contemplated to address the unique needs of children who might be accidentally caught up in a major disaster or intentionally targeted, say, in a terrorist attack?"

The panel members up in the front looked at each other and chattered among themselves. Then the moderator spoke.

"Well, I guess I need to let you know that, honestly, the issue of how to protect children has never been formally discussed, at least to the best of our knowledge. And if none of us is aware of any such discussion, I would conclude that it hasn't happened."

Later that afternoon, I called a friend, Dr. Louis Cooper, a well-respected leader in the American Academy of Pediatrics, and told him about the conversation at the briefing.

"What do you suggest?" Lou asked.

"We need a formal process in the Academy to begin planning strategies to make sure that the needs of children are on the table. How does 'The Task Force on Terrorism' sound?"

"Perfect!" Lou said. "I'll get on it tomorrow."

So, in what may be the quickest response ever seen at the stodgy offices of the venerable American Academy of Pediatrics, the task force was established and began its work with—for a big bureaucratic organization—lightning speed.

On a more personal level, my son Michael, then twenty-five years old and still working on figuring out what he was going to do with his life, along with his girlfriend Ania Wajnberg, a medical student at the Albert Einstein College of Medicine, volunteered to help distribute supplies to the workers on the still burning pile. After a few days, Michael called me.

"Dad, I figured it out."

"Meaning, exactly what?" I asked.

"I'm going to med school. I want to be able to do more than hand out water bottles to people in need."

"I get it, of course. And did that beautiful, brilliant med student girlfriend of yours have anything to do with your decision?"

"You'll never know."

"Whatever. I am proud of you, sonny boy."

And in a flash of years, on a beautiful spring day in 2007, I experienced the indescribable joy of placing the medical school graduation hood over the big shoulders of my son, now Michael Aaron Redlener, MD.

Meanwhile, in my role as president of the Children's Hospital at Montefiore and still president of the Children's Health Fund, I established a new Pediatric Preparedness program, and it was off to the races. In short order, I hired a real subject matter expert in this field, Dr. David Markenson. The two of us began writing grants, setting up protocols, and making policy recommendations that would help make sure that the needs of children at risk in disasters would be understood and accommodated.

Two years later, Alan Rosenfield invited me to lunch, "just to catch up," he said. Not quite true. He asked if I would consider coming to Columbia and leading the Mailman School's effort to establish a major program on disaster preparedness. Karen and I discussed the offer and its implications at great length.

Ultimately it seemed like the thing to do, and in April 2003, while I maintained a full schedule as president of CHF, I moved my academic appointment from Montefiore and the Albert Einstein College of Medicine to Columbia University. This was a real growth opportunity and a chance to focus on an area to which I had long been attracted: trying to make America less vulnerable to any disaster, including natural catastrophes or major industrial and infrastructure failures, as well as terrorism. The nation needed to understand and enhance its overall state of resiliency, and I looked forward to helping define what all this meant, under a new enterprise we called the National Center for Disaster Preparedness (NCDP) at Columbia University.

A critical aspect of this work for me was about the special vulnerabilities of children who were already "high risk" well before any disaster actually hit. These were poor children who lived with reduced access to health care, transportation, or good schools—a range of opportunity disparities. These are the children who will be most at risk in and after a disaster, whose communities will struggle most at the time and in the process of recovery.

That reality got played out in bright relief just two years later when the monster Hurricane Katrina and the failure of the flood levees wrecked much of the city of New Orleans. It was precisely the poorest neighborhood, the Lower Ninth Ward, where the most devastation occurred. Thousands of homes and businesses were destroyed. Medical clinics and medical records were gone. Children in the middle of chemotherapy for cancer were transported to facilities out of state without records of what medications they were on or what protocols were being followed.

Both the Children's Health Fund and the new National Center for Disaster Preparedness responded immediately to this megadisaster. Paul Simon, Karen, and I were at the Gulf within three days of Katrina's landfall and the collapse of the levee system.

By the time we arrived, the two mobile clinics I had deployed from CHF's national network were already on-site, initially in the middle of massive destruction in Gulfport-Biloxi, Mississippi. Ultimately, scores of CHF medical staff and at least seven mobile clinics rotated in and out of the area to help in the massive relief efforts that had to be mounted. Meanwhile, NCDP had begun helping states assess the needs of families and children most affected by the disaster and demoralized by the long, highly inefficient recovery from the widespread destruction brought by Hurricane Katrina.

For both organizations, it was all hands on deck. Everybody was working seven days a week, making sure that we were doing everything we could to help in the rescue and recovery efforts. Even Michael Redlener and his (almost) fiancée, Ania, were dispatched to work on our mobile units and do their part as clinicians. Stephanie Redlener, then a twenty-five-year-old marketing and communications expert with a brilliant mind for complex logistics, showed up at CHF headquarters and helped locate mobile medical units that we could deploy in the rescue efforts that were in full swing.

Meanwhile, the Columbia center got grant support to organize and implement a comprehensive and sustained tracking system for how children fared under recovery efforts throughout the region. The results of the tracking showed that thousands of children suffered long-term health and mental health consequences from a disorganized recovery process, still incomplete in 2016, that failed to recognize or meet the needs of the region's poorest children and their struggling families.

Thousands of New Orleans's most economically disadvantaged citizens were literally warehoused in the city's cold and under-resourced Superdome. Children and parents became separated, and fear was everywhere. Schools were closed or destroyed, as were many clinics. Even death counts for people from the poorer areas of New Orleans were inaccurately tracked and tabulated.

Unsure of what to do with so many poor families, Louisiana and the federal government cooperated in the development of clusters of shelters away from New Orleans, many in Baton Rouge. One of the more notorious of these "recovery communities" was called Renaissance Village. It was a cluster of some 500 newly built, very small travel trailers, all contained within a high chain-link fence, with "security and control" being managed by a Haliburton off-shoot, staffed by tough guys in khaki cargo pants and dark shirts. Think minimum security prison.

Although Oprah built a lovely recreation center and playground at Renaissance Village, life was miserable for the families assigned there. Renaissance Village was totally isolated. Finding and securing employment were difficult for parents, and access to schools or health care for children was particularly challenging. That why Children's Health Fund placed and maintained a full-service mobile pediatric clinic on the premises until Renaissance Village was eventually shut down, some eighteen months after it was opened.

To add to this unfortunate, essentially botched recovery for the most vulnerable families stuffed into those 250-square-foot trailers, a terrible discovery was later made public. FEMA's intentions were good, and all of the trailers were new, but it seems that the glue used to assemble the trailers was not given a sufficient time to "cure." So, for months the glue emitted high levels of formaldehyde, a neurotoxic agent especially dangerous for children. We and a few other organizations raised hell about this additional insult to the well-being of children and families. The CDC committed to getting baseline levels of formaldehyde and was supposed to follow affected children for the next ten years. There is no evidence that that actually ever happened.

As with so many other issues I have dealt with as a physician-advocate, there are many ways to help inform and educate the public, manage media, and influence policy makers. Every successful advocacy effort magnifies the impact of our day-to-day work. Yes, I have been creating programs to improve America's disaster resiliency and response or recovery competency, but the quantifiable impact of these programs is limited to relatively small numbers of individuals and communities. Getting the American Academy of Pediatrics to create a new task force designed to elucidate the pediatrician's role in dealing with the consequences of terrorism or other disasters has a much wider influence on so many more children.

And from 2009 through April of 2011, I served on a ten-person National Commission on Children and Disasters, chaired by the charismatic Mark Shriver, son of Eunice Kennedy and Sargent Shriver. All of the commissioners were appointed by the president or the leaders of the two Houses of Congress. We studied reports, deliberated, and summoned individuals to testify. By the time the commission was set to expire, we submitted a summary report with explicit recommendations to relevant federal agencies, all strongly suggesting policy and procedural processes crafted to ensure that the needs of children were officially and sufficiently incorporated into disaster planning across the federal government. These policies remain in place as motivators and guidelines to define how to ensure that children's needs before, during, and after a major disaster are part of the planning process at every level of government.

The takeaway here is that there are many ways to influence policy making with the goal of ensuring that people are paying attention to the needs of children. For people busy with their careers, families, and other important priorities, organizations can act as surrogates for interested, busy advocates. Parent-Teacher Associations, the medical specialty societies, and civic groups can often advocate on your behalf on the issues you are concerned about.

Presidential Politics

By the middle of 1991, my relationship with then Democratic senator Jay Rockefeller of West Virginia had become close. He was one of the congressional leaders pushing hard to create a health care system built on the principles of universal access to affordable care. He was also one of the senators whom Paul Simon and I met during our visits to the Capitol, seeming to be clearly excited about what CHF was doing for children, an issue he cared deeply about in his own work as an activist legislator and policy wonk.

Even among his own esteemed and highly accomplished family members going back three generations, Jay stood out. His career was essentially about public service, with a rapid rise through West Virginia state political offices culminating in the governorship before being elected to serve as U.S. senator from 1985 to 2015. Rockefeller, one of the few Democrats in his family, was always a true activist and a doer, leading key Senate committees and articulating strong positions on issues ranging from health care to intelligence and foreign affairs. So when he declared himself a candidate for the U.S. presidency, nobody was surprised, and many, myself included, were thrilled at the prospect. I signed up to help in the campaign and had an opportunity to travel with him as a volunteer, still actively involved in developing CHF as my critically engaging "day job."

After a few months, though, the senator opted out, presumably not finding the business of mounting and sustaining a national campaign the best way to spend his considerable energy. He returned to the Senate as a trusted leader, finally retiring in January 2015.

I wondered why and how this national scion ended up in West Virginia. It seems that after graduating from college in 1961, Rockefeller had secured a position in Washington, DC, as an assistant to the founding director of the Peace Corps, Sargent Shriver—Mark's father—recommended for the job by Bobby Kennedy, then U.S. attorney general. But Rockefeller didn't confine himself to a desk job in Washington. He served first in the Peace Corps posted to the Philippines, then joined VISTA (Volunteers in Service to America), the domestic version of Peace Corps. Assigned to Emmons, West Virginia, Rockefeller worked hard to make sure that residents of that impoverished community in one of America's poorest states had opportunities to get needed services, including health care, education, and jobs. As Jay pointed out repeatedly, he was using mobile units to provide health care screening for rural West Virginia long before we dreamed up the Children's Health Fund and developed of our own fleet of mobile units more than twenty years later.

No wonder that we hit it off. For years Rockefeller served as cochair of CHF's corporate council, and when we opened a project in Huntington, West Virginia, it was Jay Rockefeller who purchased and donated its first mobile pediatric clinic.

When Rockefeller decided to abandon his personal quest for the White House—though I think he would have made a great president—he introduced me to one of his Senate colleagues and friends, Senator Bob Kerrey of Nebraska. Kerrey was getting ready to announce his own run for the presidency.

"You'll like him," Rockefeller said. "He's really smart, very knowledgeable across just about all the major issues, and one of the main leaders around here on health system reform." That I already knew. Kerrey, the legislating iconoclast (in a good way), was influential and outspoken and, to my thinking, on the enlightened side of the issues that mattered. For a few heady months, until Kerrey, too, withdrew, I was a principal adviser for him on health care, again as a volunteer.

So that left me a twice-disappointed would-be political volunteer without a candidate. That is until my friend Dr. Steve Gleason had an idea. Steve, a family doctor from Des Moines, Iowa, was obsessively attracted to high-end politics. He had worked for presidential candidates, including Michael Dukakis in 1988. Eventually Steve had become chief of staff to Iowa governor Tom Vilsack and ultimately director of the Iowa Department of Health. But he always had his hand in presidential politics.

"Irwin, I've got something for you to think about," he said in a phone call in January of 1992. "You need to join me on the Clinton campaign. It's going to happen."

"Tell me more, Steve." And he did just that for about fifteen minutes straight.

Gleason and I had been working together for the past couple of years, organizing doctors for health reform, recruiting many into the political process, holding debates, and doing whatever else we could do to help move issues and candidates forward. On one occasion in late 1991, we organized a health care panel of all the active candidates, inviting Democrats and Republicans to come to Des Moines and say whatever they wished about the state of health care in the United States and what they would do as president.

California governor Jerry Brown, Bob Kerrey, former Massachusetts senator Paul Tsongas, and the young Arkansas governor Bill Clinton were all actively campaigning. Rhetoric and generalities characterized the comments of all of the men still in the race—except for one.

Bill Clinton stood up at the podium and looked for a moment directly into the faces of many of us in the audience. He smiled and thanked the hosts—Governor Vilsack, other local officials, Gleason, and me.

"Ladies and gentlemen. I am very pleased to be here, and I am anxious to let you know what I think about health care in America and what I think, what I know, needs to get done to fix a broken and unaffordable system. America can and must do better."

And then for forty-five minutes straight (we had asked for no more than ten minutes per speaker!), Bill Clinton talked about health care and the difference between insurance and actual access to medical services. He talked in detail about health systems in other parts of the world and how we should learn from these experiences as we developed America's unique solutions. He talked about the costs and financing of health care and eliminating disparities in access.

Clinton talked and talked, way longer than we had planned, and, needless to say, threw the whole schedule off. But he spoke with clarity and with great authority, much like a sophisticated lecture in a graduate school program. His talk was coherent and organized.

Steve leaned over to me at what turned out to be a bit past the halfway mark.

"I can't believe this. Should we try to stop him?" he asked.

"No!" I said. "This is incredible. I've never heard anything like this level of detail and deep understanding of an issue by *anybody* running for president. And do you see those notes he's reading from?"

"What notes?" Steve responded. "He doesn't have any notes."

"Exactly," I said. "The man is doing this without notes, without a net."

While the drawling, lip-biting, smooth-talking brainiac governor from Hope, Arkansas, spoke, the audience response seemed a bit tepid, perhaps a little restless. But after the event, more people crowded around him than any of the other candidates. When I finally got to him, I took the opportunity to offer some entirely unsolicited advice.

"Governor Clinton, that was a terrific talk, but with all due respect, would you consider preparing a shorter version for events like this?"

He smiled at me and said something benign before slipping away with an aide.

I watched him head out of the venue, escorted by two aides, both carrying armloads of paperwork, and all I could think of was this charming, brilliant policy wonk could actually be president. And from that moment, I was hooked, partnering with Gleason and working like crazy to get this man elected. Once in the White House, one of Bill Clinton's first actions was to appoint his wife, Hillary Rodham, to chair a major task force to develop what they hoped would be a signature accomplishment, a reformed health care system that would result in every American having accessible and affordable health care.

Ira Magaziner, a close friend of the Clintons and a brilliant consultant, was hired to run the task force. But Hillary, chair of the enterprise, remained actively involved, attending daily meetings and pushing task force members to make sure every concern was raised and every problem addressed.

Steve Gleason called me shortly after Hillary's role and the task force were announced. He had been invited to join the effort and chair the Health Professionals Review Committee, and he needed help. I was eager to do it, of course, but it was a critical time for the Children's Health Fund, and this would, in any case, be something I couldn't do without real buy-in from Karen, now running CHF's operations.

Karen did agree, though reluctantly. I'd have to move temporarily to DC, and a lot of my CHF responsibilities would fall to her. There were also more general issues, call it a diffuse discomfort, about my being away. Nonetheless, I took the position as vice chair of Steve's committee and found a hotel residence arrangement near the White House. By the beginning of February, I had thoroughly immersed myself in the utterly unique experience of working on a major initiative in a new, highly energized administration that seemed to think that anything was possible, including convincing Congress, the media, and the American people to accept a complete rebuilding of the U.S. health care system.

It didn't quite work out that way. The proposed plan, called the Health Security Act (HSA), was laid out in a 1,300-page document that became a symbol for the opposition, simply because it was very long and detailed. (If they only knew that Barack Obama's 2010 Affordable Care Act would double that length!)

Too complicated, they said of Hillary's plan. Un-American! And, they alleged, the whole process was a rigged, closed-door, secretive insiders' game. There may have been issues to criticize, aspects of the proposal that needed to be revised or rethought, but the idea of this being a closed process was patent nonsense. Not only was I there and witness to the huge numbers of people involved in the overall process, but Gleason and I were directly responsible for bringing in literally hundreds of health professionals, from nurses and hospital leadership to physicians, ancillary health professionals, and administrators from every conceivable sector of health care. They were invited to review the plans, make comments, suggest changes, and make sure they ended up being comfortable with the HSA and what it could offer the public and health providers of every stripe.

This was far from easy—and the pushback was tough to take sometimes. I asked Hillary to join a meeting I had organized with leaders of the American Academy of Pediatrics and the American Academy of Family Physicians. One question on the table was "How many well-child and prevention visits should be in the standard benefit package as part of the HSA?" That was it, a simple question. But apparently not that simple. The AAP was pushing for eight visits per year, and the family doctors thought six would do. Would they compromise at seven? No way!

Hillary was flabbergasted. I was embarrassed for my profession. After the meeting, I asked Hillary if she would consider just focusing on universal health insurance coverage for children initially, including adults later. Looking back on that moment, the timing for that kind of query was not good. Hillary was "pedal to the metal" on reforming the whole system. When that didn't work the way she hoped, she did, finally, in 1997, work with Senators Ted Kennedy, Democrat from Massachusetts, and Orin Hatch, Republican from Utah, to create the Child Health Insurance Program, or CHIP. But in the middle of the battle to reform the whole system, Hillary was not about to let up and retreat to a smaller goal. And I couldn't blame her.

One of the stranger realities of working in the White House as a volunteer was that I was "reporting" to young staffers more or less in the same age range as my own kids. Some days I had a seat or a small cubicle; some days I didn't. To my friends back home, it was exciting and just cool for me to be working at the

White House with the new president and first lady. True enough, it was all of that. But they would have been shocked to see what that meant in terms of structure, positioning, and hierarchy that affected me—and others like me. Trying to maintain the perception of myself as an experienced physician soon to turn fifty was a challenge indeed.

My friend Gleason stuck with the political work he so loved. People liked and trusted him, and his relationships with the Clintons, Senator Tom Harkin, Governor Vilsack in Iowa, and many other leaders grew. He said he wanted to do this kind of work for the rest of his life.

And he said this to me many times over the years: "I'd rather be dead than irrelevant." I never liked hearing that, mostly because I knew that he truly meant it.

Steve Gleason also carried a burden that few knew about. He had become addicted to opioid pain medications while being treated for a serious injury. He was discovered and banned from practicing medicine for five years. He recovered, and he relapsed.

In March of 2006, my dear friend, my political brother-in-arms, took his own life at a tension-filled family gathering in his Des Moines home. He had borne more sadness and grief than we knew.

I often think about how pleased Steve would have been that, although the love of his political life, Hillary Clinton, would never be elected president, major health reform was promoted and passed by President Obama in 2010. And he would have been happy to know that Clinton served so admirably as Obama's secretary of state.

On the other hand, Hillary's failed 2016 campaign for the presidency of the United States would have been as shocking and surreal to Steve as it was to me and most of the people I knew. Karen and I were thinking about attending the intended celebratory party at New York City's Javits Center. We decided to stay at home and watch the results on TV, just the two of us. Mostly we wanted to hear Hillary's acceptance speech, claiming victory over the outlandish candidacy of Donald Trump. Instead we watched in dismay as swing state after swing state turned out for the Republican outlier who had turned politics into a tour de force for off-the-wall political positions, Twitter mania, and a rhetorical coarseness unprecedented in America political history.

Three days after the election, I was scheduled to be in DC to start working on "president-elect" Hillary Clinton's transition team. That was not to be. Monday morning quarterbacking and unending hand-wringing produced multiple hypotheses as to why Clinton had to concede the election. The fact is that she definitively lost the Electoral College tally, even as she decisively prevailed in the popular contest by a margin of nearly 3 million votes over her improbable rival.

I had a personal stake in this election, too. For months I had been working as a volunteer with the campaign, helping to plan messages in a couple of areas consistent with my own expertise and experience, particularly children's issues, health care, and disaster readiness. This amounted to writing columns in swing-state newspapers, making some limited TV appearances, and, from time to time, "making suggestions." I thought that putting local doctors out as surrogates for Clinton in critical counties to support her position on health care would have been effective. The campaign disagreed.

Just a few days before the election, when the Trump campaign decided to go all out to attack Obama's (and Hillary's) Affordable Care Act, I suggested that we immediately organize a press conference with doctors and health policy professionals to forcefully refute the inaccurate allegations being made by Trump and his surrogates about "Obamacare." They certainly considered my recommendations, but the Clinton campaign twice wrote back to me emphasizing they were "staying on message" until the end. And the message was all about attacking Trump's general credibility. So the other team got a free ride attacking—with little merit—a signature position of Hillary Clinton's campaign. Who knows what mattered in the end. Whatever the real reasons for the outcome—and there were many, of course—Hillary Clinton had to absorb a painful Electoral College loss that should never have happened.

That was the end of my involvement in presidential politics, at least as far as I could predict in early 2017. It was always my perspective that leadership at the highest ranks of the government would set the tone, establish the priorities, and propose the budgets that would—or would not—focus on the issues that advocates for children feel so passionately about. In this time of confusion and uncertainty in a new administration, the likes of which we have never seen before, it's hard to know what will emerge and how it will affect America's most vulnerable children.

PART IV

Going Forward: Government, Moonshots, and Parents

The Role of Government and the
Impact of Investing in Children

While the case for a compassionate, humane focus on the well-being of children should be sufficient to make sure that our youngest citizens are properly cared for in a highly developed society, there are competing interests and economic realities that sometimes hinder this perspective. Fair enough. We do need to stimulate the economy, develop affordable housing, support the military, fight terrorism, reduce unemployment, control climate change, and so on.

But investing in children can also be seen in financial terms as a powerful means of ensuring America's continued economic strength and global influence through the twenty-first century. Here's the hard truth: we don't need more research or more data. We don't need any additional information beyond what we already know.

Who still needs to be convinced that America must protect its children, nurture their dreams and aspirations, and provide success pathways for every child? If we don't do these things, we will pay a steep and very unfortunate price over the coming decades. All of this we already know. But, one more time, let's just review what we know and what we should do, in case some of us haven't been paying attention.

The intent of child investment policies should be to:

- Maximize the resiliency and well-being of the next generations of Americans;
- Maximize the possibility of every child's fulfilling aspirations that lead to meaningful work and contributions to the tax base;
- Minimize the need for costly remediation of *preventable* challenges that lead to suboptimal development, costly physical and mental health conditions, the need for public assistance, and high rates of incarceration.

A range of America's most respected researchers have reached a number of insights and conclusions that illuminate why it is in our national interest to make sustained, evidence-informed strategic investments in our children, especially those who live in persistent poverty—and the earlier, the better. Of course parents, families, and communities have critical roles to play in ensuring that children grow up healthy, ready to learn, and ready for life—but government, too, must support families, and programs that assist them, in ways that will pay off for the nation's future.

For instance, here is the main takeaway of a 2006 Columbia University study: "Every additional high school graduate yields a net economic benefit to the public of $127,000 with benefits that are 2.5 times greater than the costs."[1] As two of the study's authors wrote in the *New York Times* in early 2012, "this is a [net] benefit to the public of nearly $90 billion for each year of success in reducing the number of high school dropouts by 700,000—or something close to $1 trillion after 11 years."[2]

A brief by Mission: Readiness and ReadyNation points out, however, that children can already be as many as eighteen months behind on milestones when they enter kindergarten.[3] Clearly, the roots of academic failure, leading to severe loss of potential to make a decent wage as an adult, begin very early in life. As I have pointed out throughout this book, understanding the trajectories of success or failure for children living with persistent adversities and disparities leads inevitably back to conditions experienced from the first day of life, if not well before, during gestation.

Noble Prize–winning economist James Heckman notes that the growing failure to acquire skills and diplomas is reducing the number of college graduates and the overall growth of the U.S. workforce; although there are "downstream" public job training programs, their impact at this later stage in the lifecycle is generally poor.[4] Similarly, the crime and court involvement so often linked to childhood disadvantage costs America $1.3 trillion per year;[5] the massive U.S. criminal justice system largely fails to "rehabilitate" adults whose disadvantage is well entrenched, and it is a huge economic cost for society.

In his acclaimed book *Enriching Children, Enriching the Nation*, economist Robert Lynch explains, "By the year 2050, the annual benefits of publicly funded universal prekindergarten would total $779 billion: $191 billion in government budget benefits, $432 billion in increased compensation of workers, and $156 billion in reduced costs to individuals from less crime and child abuse. These annual benefits in 2050 would exceed the costs of the program in that year by a ratio of 8.2 to 1."[6] He also notes that "a voluntary, high-quality, publicly funded, *universal* prekindergarten education program serving all three- and four-year-olds would begin to outstrip its annual costs within nine years and would do so by a growing margin every year thereafter."

In a related brief on programs targeting children living in poverty, Lynch concludes, "the projected government-wide budget gain from early childhood development would be 0.25 percent of GDP in 2050, about one fifth of the projected 1.27 percent of GDP deficit projected in the Social Security system for that year. This contribution toward the fiscal balance would start in less than two decades and would be achieved without raising taxes on anyone or cutting benefits for anyone."[7]

Many health conditions that disproportionately affect poor children and run rampant in disadvantaged communities have a cascading impact on both the children and their families. The prevalence and impact of asthma in children illustrates the point. Approximately 9 percent of American children, across all demographic groups, have been diagnosed with this very common chronic illness. But among poor children, the incidence of asthma is at least 50 percent higher than the national average and is thought to be the most common cause of pediatric hospital admissions.[8] For the millions of children who are homeless or living in extreme poverty, asthma rates can soar to 30 percent or more.

It is important to emphasize that these are not just dry statistics. Every child with undiagnosed or undertreated asthma represents an array of challenges that are particularly difficult for children and their families. Even finding an accessible, affordable, and good-quality doctor or clinic is a challenge for some children, especially those living in communities with persistent health care provider shortages or a lack of affordable public transportation.

When asthma is not properly controlled, children experience chronic respiratory distress, making concentrating in class or studying at home difficult, to say the least. When the asthma "attacks" become severe, an urgent trip to an emergency room—itself a terrifying experience—is necessary. Even getting to the doctor's office for checkups, so that asthma control can be fine-tuned, is challenging for families in which the breadwinner has little flexibility in terms of time off from work.

And then there are the costs to the health care system of uncontrolled asthma. With every rushed trip to the emergency room, every time a child is admitted to the hospital, costs for health care increase. This is particularly vexing for childhood asthma because total control of symptoms is possible using currently available medications. In other words, if all asthmatic children actually received standard and appropriate care, ER trips and hospital care for asthma could be virtually eliminated. Children would be listening and learning in inner-city classrooms, instead of struggling to breathe.

As mentioned earlier, the economic impact of assuring proper care would be enormous. A study by Children's Health Fund (CHF) showed that proper treatment of asthma in children dramatically reduces emergency room visits and hospitalization, reducing the cost of care by approximately $4,500 each year, on average, for every child with asthma.[9]

Another study looking at routine childhood immunization among all babies born in the United States in 2009 estimated that these immunizations will prevent some "42,000 early deaths and 20 million cases of disease, with net savings of $13.5 billion in direct costs and $68.8 billion in total societal costs, respectively."[10]

The long-term return—or, as I prefer to think of it, the positive long-term impact of smart investments in programs to support the health, education, and well-being of children—is essentially indisputable. Robert Lynch projects that "in addition to the budget savings, by the year 2050, a voluntary, high-quality, universal prekindergarten education program is estimated . . . to reduce the costs to individuals of crime and child abuse by $156 billion."[11] He also notes that investment in early childhood development for children in poverty would lower criminal justice system costs by nearly "$77 billion (or $28 billion in 2004 dollars) in 2050."

A 2008 report from the Robert Wood Johnson Foundation concluded: "A cost-benefit analysis of the Perry Preschool program estimated that approximately 80 percent of the monetary benefits of the program are benefits to the general public, with the remaining 20 percent accruing to the individual children/and or the adults they will become."[12]

In summarizing economist Robert G. Lynch's work on the benefits of early childhood education, the National Education Association observed: "Prekindergarten investments present much higher returns than the stock market. A Federal Reserve Bank of Minneapolis (2003) study determined that the total annual real rates of return (adjusted for inflation) on public investments in the Perry Preschool program exceeded 16 percent. The highly touted real rate of return on the stock market that prevailed between 1871 and 1998 was just 6.3 percent."[13]

As reported by the Children's Defense Fund, "Every year that we keep children in poverty costs our nation half a trillion dollars in lost productivity, poorer health and increased crime."[14] The 2008 Robert Wood Johnson report concluded, "Children who participate in early childhood development programs are more likely to be healthy, have higher earnings, and are less likely to commit crime and receive public assistance."[15]

Despite the clear cost-benefit logic of investing in children, a point made repeatedly by highly respected nonprofit entities like First Focus, the United States is currently going in the wrong direction. In fact, recent sequestration cuts slashed funding to children's programs by $4.2 billion in 2013.[16] The Urban Institute projects that the share of spending on children will decrease from 10 to 8 percent over the next ten years.[17] According to Bruce Lesley of First Focus, "Interest on the national debt will soon eclipse all federal investments in our nation's children combined"—despite polling that shows that "72 percent of Americans prioritize protecting investments in children equally or more than reducing the federal deficit."[18]

Many factors are essential to ensuring that every child has a chance to succeed. These include the support of parents and guardians, access to quality health care, the elimination of barriers to learning, good educational opportunities, and the mitigation of financial barriers that impede the ability of children to fulfill their aspirations.

This is not just about compassion, though that should drive everything. This is about a true "return on investment"—or maybe "impact of investment"—and doing what's right for the country's future. If we wish to ensure America's continued economic strength and global influence through the twenty-first century, we must have the discipline to make informed and appropriate investments in the nation's children.

Moonshots

I am a fan of moonshots—big bodacious efforts to solve major problems and reach cultural or scientific milestones. That's what President Obama had in mind when he announced at his last State of the Union Message, delivered to Congress in January 2016, his intention to set the nation on a course to finding cures for cancer. He asked Vice President Joe Biden to lead this effort, utilizing every resource at the nation's disposal, including all relevant expertise in government, the private sector, and academia. The very language of moonshots and huge goals is inherently exciting and motivating.

What about applying this strategy to fixing major social and economic challenges—for instance, transforming a major urban community? Can this be done?

Prospect Avenue in New York City's South Bronx is a main thoroughfare in America's poorest urban zip code. Bodegas, mom-and-pop shops, and tenements still predominate, although newly constructed townhomes, apartment buildings, and a smattering of new businesses are now appearing in a neighborhood once so notorious that the local police station was known as "Fort Apache." That was not a complimentary nod to the Old West. The station was perceived by its own officers as a fortress, a safe zone, isolated from the community, surrounded by deadly violence, crime, and ubiquitous urban decay.

241

In 1993, Fort Apache was replaced by a modern new building, just in time to help usher in the slo-mo renaissance of the South Bronx. That same year, CHF opened a storefront clinic, the South Bronx Children's Health Center. It was the first new health care program in that neighborhood in thirty years. Three years later, a modern Police Athletic League center was opened on Longwood Avenue, just two blocks from the police station, a block from the children's clinic. Ever so slowly, wrecked buildings and smoldering, debris-filled empty lots were replaced by new buildings and community services. By 2011, CHF had built three more facilities: a family clinic, a special clinic for homeless kids, and a state-of-the-art comprehensive health center called the Center for Child Health and Resiliency, affiliated with the long-standing and highly supportive Montefiore Health Center.

Of course, it's not just the CHF that has been evolving in the Bronx. Between 1980 and 2012, the borough's population grew by 240,000 people, and by 2013 total private sector wages (in constant dollars) reached their highest point in history at $9.3 billion a year. Serious crime rates have fallen by an incredible 75 percent since 1990, and more than 100,000 living units have been renovated or created. There are now some 26 percent more businesses in the Bronx than there were twenty-five years ago.[19]

While still poor and struggling with social and economic adversities, racial disparities, and the need for even more growth and better access to services, the Bronx is undeniably a community on the move. Where there was once mostly an urban nightmare, there is new cause for genuine hope.

All of these changes reflect a commitment to renewal; these antidotes to a mistaken sense of intractable hopelessness and despair are cause for at least a muted celebration of possibility realized. Zip code 10459 is still one of America's most destitute communities, but progress is real and visible—just excruciatingly slow.

Why so slow? The South Bronx was the poster child for the massive decline of American cities in the late 1970s. Nobody thought that those conditions should be tolerated—not politicians, and certainly not the residents. Eventually, after a series of what can be best characterized as random acts of investment and development projects, progress is visible. But the bottom line is that after sixty years of chaos and squalor, along with solid data to support evidence of positive change, this neighborhood remains an impoverished back alley of a great global city.

The explanation for this pitiful pace of change is, as is always the case, a combination of resources, priorities, politics, and, although it is probably less pronounced than in other struggling American cities, an element of urban segregation. Progress is being made in the South Bronx, but, for better or worse, it is not really gentrifying. There are very few blocks where middle-class white families and young commuters into Manhattan are finding the latest low-rent haven. For some that's good. The cost of living remains affordable for low-income families, but the social price paid by the residents of the South Bronx is persistent isolation from the economics, the culture, and the growth of the city as a whole. Changing this state of affairs is certainly possible, but it would take focus and resources on a grand scale. It would mean a serious commitment, an operational timeline, and leadership.

Still, it could be done. It's just that there seems to be little appetite, locally or nationally, to take on a project of such magnitude. Schools would have to be repaired physically and upgraded academically, far more decent and affordable housing would be necessary, along with more child care, senior care, cultural opportunities, parks, recreation centers—and most important, good paying jobs that would elevate families to a middle-class life.

It's not as though America is incapable of setting and meeting big goals, missions of great national priority. The nation once led the world in its capacity to dream big, plan effectively, and "make it happen," doing so competently and with a sense of urgency—precisely what is needed to truly bring the South Bronx roaring into the twenty-first century.

Massive development projects in the 1930s, like the building of the Hoover Dam and the Tennessee Valley Authority economic stimulus project, were conceived and completed at lightning speed compared with the grinding pace of creating and following through on a big idea during the past twenty years. Think about Boston's Central Artery/Tunnel Project, affectionately known as the "Big Dig." Planning for this major project began in 1982, construction began in 1991, and it was finally completed in 2007—that's a quarter century, for those keeping score. Cost overruns were spectacular, as much as 200 percent over original projections.

But massive cost overruns and long delays have not always been the reality for the nation's capacity to conceive and complete major construction projects. In the 1940s, America created an unprecedented military force that defeated powerful aggressors in World War II. In 1956, President Dwight D. Eisenhower decided that the nation needed a functional interstate highway system and convinced politicians of every stripe to make that happen. In the tumultuous 1960s, on May 25, 1961, President John F. Kennedy made a historic speech to Congress in which he declared that America must accelerate its space exploration efforts and put a man on the moon by the end of the decade. And so it was that Neil Armstrong set foot on the moon on July 21, 1969.

America's history is rife with illustrations of our ability to effectively meet enormous challenges. So, again, why do the South Bronx, Central Brooklyn, and so many other marginalized neighborhoods in so many American cities languish in poverty, racial discrimination, social strife, and violent discord?

The big picture for communities "in waiting" for rehabilitation, and for the children who live in these neighborhoods, remains distressingly pessimistic.

One-fifth of America's children live in poverty, and more than 16 million children go hungry for a significant portion of the year.[20] In 2006, about 1.5 million children experienced homelessness for some portion of the year; by 2013, that number had risen to 2.5 million.[21]

There are those who acknowledge that these are serious problems and eventually we'll need to address all of them but, at the same time, might be thinking, "In the greater scheme of things, does it really matter if rebuilding the nation's many versions of the South Bronx in persistently depressed neighborhoods, from Miami and Boston to Chicago, Detroit, Indianapolis, and Los Angeles, takes thirty years, or perhaps fifty years, instead of ten? In the big sweep of history, what seems like forever from today's vantage point may be ultimately inconsequential. Maybe we need to be patient."

Well, actually not. Patience is far from a virtue when it comes to dealing with adversities that can have a lifetime of consequences. The whole idea of "patience" is incompatible with the urgency needed to solve challenges that are highly time-sensitive for children during the years when young brains are developing, emotional health is being established, and the substrates of long-term physical health are on the line. Like families, communities need to nurture the health and well-being of children—which is why upgrading neighborhoods and supporting children in every neighborhood should be considered America's most compelling challenge.

Parenting and the Rest of Us: What We Can Do to Advance the Success of Every Child

Let me be blunt about two perspectives on the critical responsibilities of parents in making sure that their children grow up healthy, educated, and ready to enter the workplace.

First of all, there is no policy, special program, pilot project, demonstration, initiative, biblical passage, or clerical directive that can replace an appropriately loving and informed parent's extraordinary influence over the long-term well-being and success of a child.

Second, there is almost no way to create pathways for all children to realize their dreams and aspirations without addressing the unjust ravages of poverty. Parents who are poor, including many who work full-time for wages too low to rise out of poverty, live in perpetual stress, facing challenges that consume their energies and deeply demoralize them. They struggle to pay the rent or buy enough nutritious food to feed their families. They are treading water, hoping for some way out of the morass of poverty.

There are many traumas, experiences, missed opportunities, barriers, and rough roads that can deter a positive trajectory for any child. But under almost any set of circumstances, resilient parents can help their children become more resilient, more capable of overcoming many adversities. What parents offer is encouragement and irreplaceable support which, as I said, no government policy can provide. But effective parental resiliency in the context of chronic poverty is extraordinarily difficult.

There is a moral problem buried in this thesis. Why should some children and parents face far more *preventable* and pernicious adversities and disparities than others? Poverty is a powerful barrier to good health and a decent education. No American child, no child born in any prosperous society, should face poverty-based consequences that can interfere with well-being and/or later productivity.

Parents of any socioeconomic stratum can potentially be powerful buffers of almost any trauma that befalls the family or the community. Even among the millions of children who are part of the ongoing global refugee crisis, there are some who will make it through relatively unscathed, even if their lives have been severely disrupted and psychologically traumatizing for an extended period of time. This is especially true if there is a protecting adult figure, particularly a parent, buffering the conditions that threaten a child, physically or otherwise.

In refugee camps or squalid urban homeless shelters, if the agencies and volunteers can make sure that basic nutrition, clean water, and somewhat secure shelter are available and stable, a buffering adult and a resilient child may have a chance to make it through, regain their collective footing, and find a path toward a productive and positive life. As the late Elie Wiesel personified in his own life story of survival through years of constant horror in the Nazi death camp at Auschwitz, it is possible to return, deeply affected perhaps, but recommitted to a life of hope and possibilities.

Raising all children successfully—that is, to fulfill *their* dreams—is our best hope for the future and the ultimate test of America's ability to regain ground and sustain its global influence. But the nation's trajectory has degenerated into fiercely partisan and ideological camps, maybe listening to but rarely hearing each other. Where's the common mission shared by every citizen and family? Perhaps the goal is clear: make sure that every child has a shot at being a success story. But how to get there is where the common goal becomes impossible to realize, often because we resort to unyielding ideological or personal positions.

As with so many other issues, finding answers to how best to nurture our children has been drawn too much along quasi-political lines. The right wants more local and individual control, the left more government programs. But from down here in the trenches, parents know this is a false choice. We need a smart, compassionate government providing basic support to vulnerable families and resources for those who need guidance and information. But good parents, capable of independent decisions in the best interests of their own children, are indispensable.

Here's a key point worth remembering: Parents are essential to maximizing a child's potential. Parents are natural adversity buffers, universally understood to have primary responsibility for their children. But parents with limited resources can't build a new school or clean up crime in the community or create accessible, good-quality health care opportunities where none exist.

These things are the responsibility of a value-based government that understands its role in establishing a future that is inclusive and productive.

Government is not a replacement for good parents, but in the absence of a responsible government, even a great parent can't ensure that his or her children have what they need to secure a fulfilled future.

Finally, whether we're parents or not, there's a role to play for each of us to do our part on behalf of our children. If we care about the future and wish the world well, if we want to make sure that America stays resilient as a prosperous, model democracy, there are many issues that need our attention. But I suggest that there is no higher priority than eliminating the barriers that keep children from achieving their dreams and reaching their full intellectual potential. Waiting fifteen or twenty years to remediate the issues that undermine success pathways for children will be too late. The damage will have been done, and the consequences are often irrevocable.

So what do we do? We can support local efforts to ensure that every child attends a capable and competent school. We can join the local school parents' organization and vote for referendums that provide needed resources to schools. Others may choose to engage with efforts to expand access to health care for all children in their town or county. Another consideration is joining a community or national organization that supports critical programs for children. Finally, every citizen must participate in elections for officials on every level of government. Make it your business to truly understand a candidate's voting record or positions on the issues regarding the provision of needed programs to assist marginalized and vulnerable children.

Whatever individuals and communities choose to do, our best hope for moving forward is to acknowledge and nurture the grand coalition of parents, voluntary organizations, and government that together have the ability to create success pathways for every child in America.

Epilogue

THE CHILDREN WE MET at the beginning of this book, William, LaTisha, Clarence, and Raymond, represent the kind of children we identify as "high risk" or vulnerable. They live under conditions that are filled with adversity and trauma. But for many, though not all, of them, there is hope—real hope. They need support from parents and government. They need inspiration and opportunity. They need good doctors, smart teachers, and safety net programs. Their parents need help and caring support as well. The point is they are not irretrievably lost—they are waiting for a pathway, a direction to follow.

When I was running the pediatric intensive care unit at the Jackson Memorial Hospital in Miami in the mid-1970s, there was one doctor I could count on consulting with at any hour of the day or night, a now retired pediatric surgeon named Marc Rowe. We'd sit in the unit going over cases, planning medical strategies, and assessing the status of every child. Marc was among the smartest, most caring physicians I had ever met.

Marc was focused and deliberate when it came to bringing children into the operating suite. He wanted to make sure medical treatment options were explored before adding the risk of surgery to a very sick, fragile child's overall condition. But when a child needed surgery, Marc took care of business. In the OR he was well known for his extraordinary skill and dexterity. More important, I could always count on his judgment, reliably clear and based on experience and scientific evidence. And there were few doctors who could communicate with patients and families with the empathy and sweetness that he could. When the chips were down, when it was showtime, Marc was the doctor you'd want by your side.

You might imagine that Marc was a straight-A student from prekindergarten through high school, perhaps valedictorian, who got a full scholarship to a top-ranked college and easy admission to medical school, right? Well, not exactly. Marc Rowe grew up literally labeled "retarded"; he attended "special classes" or had special accommodations in a regular classroom. He had severe learning disabilities involving reading, writing, comprehension, and computational skills. He was headed to welding school after high school until a friend and fellow athlete convinced him that he should go to college. He did—and ultimately became one of the world's greatest pediatric surgeons.

The point here is that children face all kinds of adversities that may seem overwhelming—impenetrable challenges that represent barriers to fulfilling aspirations and realizing dreams. For most of the children I have seen in more than forty years of working with families who live in extreme social and economic stress, dreams are dreamt but are soon extinguished by conditions over which they have little control.

Other children never have a chance, growing up in isolated environments where even the process of understanding what *might* be possible is too obscure, where expectations are profoundly depressed. Sometimes the potential in a child is tragically just missed by his teachers, his family, and his community. That is often the case among children I've seen who may have had a health or behavioral issue that obscured keen underlying intelligence or impeded academic performance. Children with unrecognized and untreated hearing or vision problems, for instance, may be labeled as underperformers and, sadly, even come to see themselves as incapable and undeserving of a big dream.

That really was Dr. Rowe's story, too, even though he was not additionally burdened by poverty, homelessness, or other social factors that keep so many children from achieving their potential.

What's important to remember are three core principles:

1. We must strive to make sure that every child's potential is recognized, understanding that it is a moral failing to deprive children of a pathway to succeed and be fulfilled. This is about social justice, human needs, and the inherent value of every individual child.

2. National objectives for the United States, as for any nation that wants to be economically successful, innovative, and influential in the world, must start with understanding that nurturing the aspirations of all of its children is essential to its future success. Children can grow up to be productive, fulfilled, and contributing citizens or become dependent, high-need, nonproductive citizens requiring remediation. We have the power to tip the balance in favor of the former goal.

3. Good parenting, child-centric policies and spending priorities, strong child-based institutions, and resilient children are the elements of a society that is optimally prepared for the future.

I'd like to end as we began, by telling you about another remarkable child I met in a clinic built to care for disadvantaged children in New York City.

Lucy was an adorable fourth grader I met in the South Bronx in 2013. She was at the clinic for a checkup, but she had a lot to say. When I asked her what she wanted to be when she grew up, she couldn't wait to tell me.

"I want to be a nurse or a teacher."

"Really. Those are both great ideas. What would you like about being a teacher or a nurse?" I asked.

"Well, they both help people, and I know I would like to help other kids."

"That's a really good reason."

"I know!" she bubbled. "Last year there was a girl in my class who came to school hungry every day."

I responded, "That's sad to hear."

"But we helped her," said Lucy. "My mom said I could invite her over for dinner after school. So we did. Every day she came home with me. Every day until the end of the year. Sometimes her mom came, too. Then they moved away."

"By the way, where do you live?" I asked.

"Well, my mom, my brother, and me live a few blocks from here—in the Prospect shelter," Lucy said, referring to a nearby *homeless* shelter.

"How long have you guys been at the Prospect?" I asked.

"For a long time. A very long time."

A heart of gold. A homeless mother and her two children opening up their room in the shelter to another child. I looked at this beautiful little girl and tried to absorb the profound compassion shown by Lucy and her family, themselves struggling, to help someone in even more need than they were.

This is a short story of compassion—something we all need to remember. Even if we understand that our *future* depends on the investments we make in the health, education, and well-being of children, the *present*, how we treat each other right now, counts a lot. In fact, it's our present that shows us who we are and why we deserve a future that's worthy of America's values and our sustained ability to make the world a better place for each and every human being on our fragile planet.

Notes

Introduction: The Urgency of Childhood

1. The Sentencing Project, *Report of the Sentencing Project to the United Nations Human Rights Committee Regarding Racial Disparities in the United States Criminal Justice System*, August 2013,http://sentencingproject.org/wp-content/uploads/2015/12/Race-and-Justice-Shadow-Report-ICCPR.pdf.

2. Emma Brown and Alejandra Matos, "Nation's High School Graduation Rate Reaches New Record High," *Washington Post*, October 17, 2016.

I. Kids Who Dream, Kids Who Can't

1. Peter Dreier, "Reagan's Real Legacy," *Nation*, February 4, 2011.

2. Roy Grant, Delaney Gracy, Grifin Goldsmith, Alan Shapiro, and Irwin E. Redlener, "Twenty-Five Years of Child and Family Homelessness: Where Are We Now?" *American Journal of Public Health* 103, Suppl. 2 (2013): e1–e10.

3. E. Fuller Torrey, "Ronald Reagan's Shameful Legacy: Violence, the Homeless, Mental Illness," *Salon.com*, September 29, 2013.

4. Drew Desilver, "Black Unemployment Rate Is Consistently Twice That of Whites," *Pew Research Center*, August 21, 2013, http://www.pewresearch.org/fact-tank/2013/08/21/through-good-times-and-bad-black-unemployment-is-consistently-double-that-of-whites/.

5. Giselle Routhier, *State of the Homeless 2016*, Coalition for the Homeless, 2016, http://www.coalitionforthehomeless.org/state-of-the-homeless-2016/.

6. Eugene M. Lewit, "Children in Foster Care," *Future of Children* 3, no. 3 (1993): 192–200.

7. Irwin Redlener, Delaney Gracy, and Dennis Walto, *Unfinished Business: More Than 20 Million Children in U.S. Still Lack Sufficient Access to Essential Health Care*, Children's Health Fund, November 2016, https://www.children shealthfund.org/wp-content/uploads/2016/11/Unfinished-Business-Final_.pdf.

8. Routhier, *State of the Homeless 2016*.

9. Jessica M. Solis, Julia M. Shadur, Alison R. Burns, and Andrea M. Hussong, "Understanding the Diverse Needs of Children Whose Parents Abuse Substances," *Current Drug Abuse Reviews* 5, no. 2 (2012): 135–147.

10. Settlement Housing Fund, "St. John's Place," 2017, http://www.settlement housingfund.org/st_johns_place.html.

11. Routhier, *State of the Homeless 2016*.

12. Centers for Disease Control and Prevention (CDC), *Data, Statistics, and Surveillance*, 2017, https://www.cdc.gov/asthma/asthmadata.htm.

13. Roy Grant, Shawn Bowen, Diane E. McLean, Douglas Berman, Karen Redlener, and Irwin Redlener, "Asthma Among Homeless Children in New York City," *American Journal of Public Health* 97, no. 3 (2007): 448–450.

14. Economic Innovation Group, *The 2016 Distressed Community Index*, 2016, http://eig.org/wp-content/uploads/2016/02/2016-Distressed-Communities -Index-Report.pdf.

15. Bureau of Health Workforce Health, Resources and Services Administration, *Shortage Areas, Health Professional Shortage Area (HPSA)—Basic Primary Medical Care*, January 1, 2017, http://datawarehouse.hrsa.gov/tools /hdwreports/Reports.aspx.

16. Roy Grant et al., *The Health Transportation Shortage Index: The Development and Validation of a New Tool to Identify Underserved Communities*. Children's Health Fund, 2012, https://issuu.com/childrenshealthfund /docs/chf_htsi-monograph__2_?mode=window.

17. Roy Grant, Shawn K. Bowen, Matthew Neidell, Timothy Prinz, and Irwin E. Redlener, "Health Care Savings Attributable to Integrating Guidelines-Based Asthma Care in the Pediatric Medical Home," *Journal of Health Care for the Poor and Underserved* 21, Suppl. 2 (2010): 82–92.

II. Roots

1. International Food Policy Research Institute, *A Visual Guide to the Future World Food Situation*, 2000, http://pdf.usaid.gov/pdf_docs/Pnacj176.pdf.

III. Real-World Medicine and Public Health

1. American Society for the Positive Care of Children, "Child Abuse Statistics," 2017, http://americanspcc.org/child-abuse-statistics/.

2. Linda T. Kohn, Janet M. Corrigan, and Molla S. Donaldson, eds., "To Err is Human: Building a Safer Health System," 1999, http://www.nationalacademies.org/hmd/Reports/1999/To-Err-is-Human-Building-A-Safer-Health-System.aspx.

3. Suzanne Franks, "Ethiopian Famine: How Landmark BBC Report Influenced Modern Coverage," *Guardian*, October 22, 2014.

4. Giselle Routhier, *State of the Homeless 2016*, Coalition for the Homeless, 2016, http://www.coalitionforthehomeless.org/state-of-the-homeless-2016/.

5. Robin Denselow, "Paul Simon's *Graceland*: The Acclaim and the Outrage," *Guardian*, April 19, 2012.

6. Carol Tannenhauser, *Cuba Notes*, unpublished manuscript, no date.

IV. Going Forward

1. Henry Levin, Clive Belfield, Peter Muennig, and Cecilia Rouse, *The Costs and Benefits of an Excellent Education for All of America's Children*. Teachers College, Columbia University, January 2007, http://cbcse.org/wordpress/wp-content/uploads/2013/03/2007-Levin.Excellent-educatin-for-all-of-america%C2%B4s-children.pdf.

2. Henry M. Levin and Cecelia E. Rouse, "The True Cost of High School Dropouts," *New York Times*, January 25, 2012.

3. Mission: Readiness and ReadyNation, *STEM and Early Childhood—When Skills Take Root*, May 2016, http://www.prekforpa.org/wp-content/uploads/2016/06/MR_RN-Skills-Gap-PA_v3.pdf.

4. See James J. Heckman, "The American High School Graduation Rate: Trends and Levels," *Review of Economics and Statistics* 92, no. 2 (2010): 244–262.

5. James J. Heckman and Dimitriy V. Masterov, "The Productivity Argument for Investing in Young Children," *Review of Agricultural Economics* 29, no. 3 (2007): 446–493.

6. Robert G. Lynch, *Enriching Children, Enriching the Nation: Public Investment in High-Quality PreKindergarten* (Washington, DC: EPI Press, 2007).

7. Robert G. Lynch, "Early Childhood Investment Yields Big Payoff," *West Ed Policy Perspectives*, 2005, https://www.wested.org/online_pubs/pp-05-02.pdf.

8. See Centers for Disease Control and Prevention (CDC), *Data, Statistics, and Surveillance*, 2017, https://www.cdc.gov/asthma/asthmadata.htm.

9. Roy Grant, Shawn K. Bowen, Matthew Neidell, Timothy Prinz, and Irwin E. Redlener, "Health Care Savings Attributable to Integrating Guidelines-Based Asthma Care in the Pediatric Medical Home," *Journal of Health Care for the Poor and Underserved* 21, Suppl. 2 (2010): 82–92.

10. Fangjun Zhou, Abigail Shefer, Jay Wenger, Mark Messonnier, Li Yan Wang, Adriana Lopez, Matthew Moore, Trudy V. Murphy, Margaret Cortese, and Lance Rodewald, "Economic Evaluation of the Routine Childhood Immunization Program in the United States, 2009," *Pediatrics* 133, no. 4 (2014): 577–585.

11. Lynch, *Enriching Children*.

12. Robert Wood Johnson Foundation, "Early Childhood Experiences: Laying the Foundation for Health Across a Lifetime," *Issue Brief 1: Early Childhood Experiences and Health*, June 2008, http://www.commissiononhealth.org/PDF/095bea47-ae8e-4744-b054-258c9309b3d4/Issue%20Brief%201%20Jun%2008%20-%20Early%20Childhood%20Experiences%20and%20Health.pdf.

13. National Education Association (NEA), "Fact Sheet: Enriching Children, Enriching the Nation," 2007, http://www.nea.org/home/18190.htm.

14. Children's Defense Fund, "End Child Poverty," 2017, http://www.childrensdefense.org/policy/policy-priorities-overviews/endchildpoverty.html.

15. Robert Wood Johnson Foundation, "Early Childhood Experiences."

16. First Focus, "Fact Sheet: Kids Lose Billions with Sequester," February 2013, https://firstfocus.org/wp-content/uploads/2013/02/FirstFocus-TaxPolicy-2013SequestrationsImpactonKids.pdf.

17. Julia B. Isaacs, Sara Edelstein, Heather Hahn, Katherine Toran, and C. Eugene Steuerle, "Kids' Share 2013: Federal Expenditures on Children in 2012 and Future Projections," Urban Institute, 2013, http://www.urban.org/sites/default/files/publication/23981/412903-Kids-Share-Federal-Expenditures-on-Children-in-and-Future-Projections.PDF.

18. Bruce Lesley, "Invest in Kids: Restoring the American Dream," *First Focus: Voices for Kids Blog*, 2014, https://firstfocus.org/blog/invest-in-kids-restoring-the-american-dream/.

19. Office of the State Comptroller, *An Economic Snapshot of the Bronx*, Report 4–2014, July 2013, https://www.osc.state.ny.us/osdc/rpt4-2014.pdf.

20. National Center for Children in Poverty (NCCP), "Child Poverty," 2017, http://www.nccp.org/topics/childpoverty.html.

21. Ellen L. Bassuk, *America's Youngest Outcasts: A Report Card on Child Homelessness*, American Institutes for Research, November 2014, http://www.air.org/sites/default/files/downloads/report/Americas-Youngest-Outcasts-Child-Homelessness-Nov2014.pdf.

Index